Eating to Lose

Healing from a Life of Diabulimia

Maryjeanne Hunt

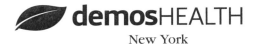

demosHEALTH

New York

Visit our website at www.demoshealth.com

ISBN: 978-1-9363-0327-4
E-book ISBN: 978-1-6170-5103-6
Acquisitions Editor: Noreen Henson
Production Editor: Michael Lisk
Compositor: Manila Typesetting Company
Printer: Hamilton Printing

Medical information provided by Demos Health, in the absence of a visit with a healthcare professional, must be considered as an educational service only. This book is not designed to replace a physician's independent judgment about the appropriateness or risks of a procedure of therapy for a given patient. Our purpose is to provide you with information that will help you make your own healthcare decisions.

The information and opinions provided here are believed to be accurate and sound, based on the best judgment available to the authors, editors, and publisher, but readers who fail to consult appropriate health authorities assume the risk of injuries. The publisher is not responsible for errors or omissions. The editors and publisher welcome any reader to report to the publisher any discrepancies or inaccuracies noticed.

Library of Congress Cataloging-in-Publication Data
Hunt, Maryjeanne.
　Eating to lose : healing from a life of diabulimia / Maryjeanne Hunt.
　　p. cm.
　　ISBN 978-1-936303-27-4 (pbk.)
　1. Diabetes—Popular works. 2. Diabetes—Diet therapy—Popular works. 3. Bulimia—Popular works. I. Title.
　RC660.H88 2012
　362.196'462—dc23
　　　　　　　　　　　　　　　　　　　　2011039056

Made in the United States of America
11 12 13 14　　5 4 3 2 1

Contents

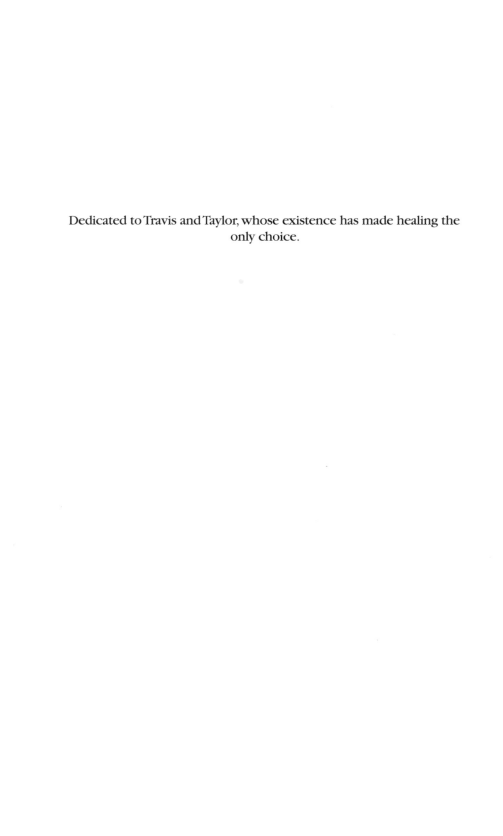

Dedicated to Travis and Taylor, whose existence has made healing the only choice.

Foreword

Research shows that approximately 30 percent of women with Type 1 Diabetes restrict insulin during their lifetimes. While a smaller percentage of these women could be diagnosed with a clinical eating disorder, women with Type 1 Diabetes have over twice the risk of developing an eating disorder than women without diabetes.

Insulin restriction is a problem unique to Type 1 Diabetes in which the patient intentionally takes less insulin than prescribed, which induces high blood sugars usually to purge calories and lose weight. Insulin restriction places patients with Type 1 Diabetes at increased risk for diabetic ketoacidosis, a medical crisis that can be fatal. It is also associated with earlier onset and higher rates of long-term medical complications of diabetes such as retinopathy, nephropathy, and neuropathy, as well as increased risk of early mortality.

In the last several years, this problem has been dubbed "Diabulimia" by the mainstream media. Mental health professionals often disagree with the use of this term and instead refer to it as the dual diagnosis of eating disorders and Type 1 Diabetes. Regardless of what we call it, media attention has helped to raise awareness of this important women's health issue. Now that patients and health care providers have a way of understanding it and terms to call it, it is my sincere hope that more of those who are struggling will be able to access appropriate help. Patients tell me that, until recently, they had no idea that others shared this problem. Too often, I have been told that even when these women tried to seek treatment, they either could not find it or that it did not address the connections between their eating disorder and their diabetes.

My treatment of these patients has taught me that recovery is possible but involves the hard work of changing their relationship with food, insulin and diabetes management, and their worries about weight. Recent research actually confirms that recovery occurs in conjunction with decreasing fears that achieving healthy blood sugar ranges will automatically result in weight gain. In fact, the women who improved their blood sugars typically stabilized their weight, while those who continued to restrict insulin often gained weight.

Eating to Lose fills an important need for women with Type 1 Diabetes, who have long felt that they were struggling alone with insulin restriction. Maryjeanne Hunt's personal story provides one more hopeful example that recovery can happen. This is her unique story about her journey toward wellness. Each woman's process will be her own, but they will all share the common goal of working hard to improve their long-term health and present-day quality of life.

Ann Goebel-Fabbri, PhD
Assistant Professor of Psychiatry
Harvard Medical School

Behavioral and Mental Health Unit
Joslin Diabetes Center
1 Joslin Place
Boston, MA 02215

Introduction

In 1980, there were fewer than six million people in the United States living with diabetes. I was one of them. I was diagnosed with the disease in 1971. By 2004, the number of Americans with diabetes had grown to nearly 16 million. Just four years later, that number climbed to 23.6 million. Today, at 25.8 million strong, the diabetes epidemic is costing our country over $200 billion dollars a year in healthcare expenses, and is expected to cost $3.4 trillion by the end of this decade, making it one of the most urgent public health issues of our time (American Diabetes Association, January 26, 2011; United Health, November 23, 2010).

Insulin is the cornerstone for treating Type 1 Diabetes. According to the American Diabetes Association, diabetic women are nearly three times more likely to develop an eating disorder than non-diabetic women. An estimated 30-40 percent of female teens and young adults with Type 1 Diabetes have developed or will develop an eating disorder. Once again, I was one of them. *Diabulimia,* as the disorder is known today, is the dangerous and often fatal practice where an individual with Type 1 Diabetes alters or omits insulin for the purpose of weight loss. I'm no mathematical genius, but it seems to me, that translates to a whole lot of American people *not* living the American Dream!

Diabetes is a disease where the pancreas, one of the body's organs, discontinues insulin production. Insulin is the body's only means of turning sugar into usable energy. No insulin means no energy—for anything from healing and growing to thinking and running. Without insulin, we cannot survive for very long. Non-diabetic people produce insulin automatically, but those with Type 1 Diabetes (Juvenile Diabetes) must inject insulin into their bodies to stay alive.

In the absence of adequate insulin, glucose (sugar) accumulates in the blood. It is necessary for our bodies to have a certain amount of sugar in our blood so that it can supply energy to the cells in our bodies as needed. A normal (non-diabetic) blood sugar range is 80 ml/dl—120 ml/dl. Since this is not a textbook, it's not necessary to know more precisely what these numbers represent, only that they are the *ideal* range.

When sugar accumulates in the blood, the non-diabetic body knows to signal the pancreas to produce appropriate amounts of insulin to keep it in the ideal range. The non-diabetic pancreas is quite intelligent and does this all on its own. When excess sugar accumulates in the blood of a person with diabetes because the dose of insulin is either insufficient or nonexistent, the diabetic body produces *ketones*, which use up the body's fat for energy at a much faster rate than calorie restriction and/or exercise.

I know what you're thinking: If you're like most women in this country who put weight loss right up there with love and money, *ketones* probably sound like a dieter's panacea! Well, they are . . . . and they're not. You see, in addition to rapid fat-loss, the body also loses muscle tissue and fluid pretty quickly too. The entire process, called *diabetic ketoacidocis*, is a potentially life-threatening condition that produces high concentrations of toxins in the blood and causes extreme vomiting and intense dehydration. Still sound like a dream-come-true?

On the other hand, when the blood sugar drops too *low*—like when a meal has been skipped or delayed, exercise was more vigorous than planned, or when the insulin dose happened to be too high for the conditions of the time—quick acting carbohydrates like table sugar, fruit juice, or candy become an urgent life-saving remedy.

Okay, that's it . . . . for now. I'm not a doctor and you're probably not studying to be one. Here's the bottom line: While most people achieve weight loss by eating *less*, I was able to achieve the same goal by eating *more*, as long as I remained 'diligent' about off-setting a binge with an omission of insulin.

COLLISION COURSE

1

Body Image Setup

The Green Dress

Mirror, mirror on the wall . . . for some of us, this not-so-innocent sheet of reflective glass draws you to it like an unkind magnet, attaching itself to you, insisting its truth upon you. It can become so connected to you that you strangely grow overprotective of its cruelty, addicted to every glimpse of imperfection it reveals. . . .

For my eighth grade self, the day this common household wall-hanging echoed back to me an image that more closely resembled a cylinder of Pillsbury crescent rolls about to burst out of their airtight packaging than a twelve-year-old girl desperate for a single morsel of affirmation, was the day it crossed over to the other side. The war between the mirror and me had begun.

I can still see that image perfectly. I had just squeezed every piece of my body into a second-hand dress I had borrowed to wear to my cousin's wedding. I can recall every single detail of that dress. How unforgiving it had been to my preadolescent body—the Kelly green jersey fabric draped down my expanding middle, the pink and black appliqué elastic struggling to clench my underdeveloped chest. It made me look so . . . so . . . Oh, what the heck, there's no other way to say it: *UGLY!*

"Mom, I hate this one! It makes me look . . . fat!" To this point, I had never been fat a day in my life. I was the one that kids made fun of for being too skinny. It had been a shocking revelation.

"You just look a little . . . ummm . . ." Mom paused to search for the right word, "chunky," she finally admitted.

Chunky! Was that supposed to make me feel *better?* What did that mean? Maybe something like, 'You're not exactly fat; you're just . . . um . . . kinda fat.' Or like, 'Let's just find a more palatable word for the truth.' Or better yet, 'Let's just bury the truth inside a whole bunch of euphemisms.'

That "truth" as I saw it would become the beginning of my education on the intimate link between food, calories, body image—and balance.

Adolescence marks a time of rapid and intense emotional and physical changes, for all children. There is an increased value placed on acceptance by friends and a heightened attention to social messages about cultural norms and body image.

The Four-Letter Word

I was a skinny child until eighth grade. Then I suppose nature decided it was about time I started to develop a few female curves. But that wasn't how I saw it. The curves seemed to happen in all the wrong places. And my developing body bore no resemblance to those perfect models in the fashion magazines and television commercials of the seventies. Why couldn't I look more like them?

But oh how privileged I was to have an in-house "expert" at my disposal. You see, through my entire childhood Mom, the world's greatest authority on dieting, ate meals that were different from the meals she served to the rest of the family. I suppose I must have surmised in my naiveté that she simply had a particular affinity for broiled fish and spinach or plain skinless chicken breast and broccoli. What other explanation could there have been for her limited menu choices while the rest of us got to feast on spaghetti and meatballs or roast beef and baked potatoes smothered in butter, or better yet, Rosetti's pizza?

But somewhere between sandboxes and prom dresses, I learned the meaning of the word "diet," and that Mom ate this way because she was always on one. She never allowed us to witness her eating dessert with the rest of us, unless of course it happened to be one of those rare occasions when she gave herself permission to "cheat" (a word that I've finally learned never belongs in the same sentence as "food"). As long as I can remember, my mom had "just five more pounds to lose." In those days, I saw her as the rock star of diet savvy. So when it was time for me to shed a few pounds, her guidance was indeed a welcome commodity.

As a fourteen-year-old with diabetes, I learned to like cottage cheese with pineapple and a few Grapenuts sprinkled over the top in place of hot fudge sundaes, and dry tuna (hold the bread) instead of burgers with the fixings. I became a walking encyclopedia of calories, fat grams, and carbs. Salad became my best friend, and hot fudge sundaes, French fries, and pizza, my enemies. And yes, if I was feeling especially underprivileged, I got to "cheat" too. And then? I got to feel guilty for days later.

D-I-E-T. It's all about The Bad List. Once you deny yourself something, you crave it—physically, mentally, or both. The whole process becomes a negative one. More focused on what you're *not* supposed to eat for the next umpteen days, weeks, or months, than what you're *allowed* to savor—guilt-free (well, at least according to *this* particular system of food regulation)—you struggle to remain faithful to your new set of eating rules.

Putting your daughter on a diet, even if she's overweight, can damage her relationship with food or distort her body image which may increase her risk of developing an eating disorder later in life.

Ah yes, the rules. NO pizza. NO brownies. NO potato chips. You love pizza and brownies and potato chips but you can give them up for just two weeks, right? Because if you do, you will lose ten pounds. And if you lose just ten pounds, you will finally be pretty enough. And pretty enough will most assuredly lead to happy enough. Of course, it's worth two weeks of no pizza and brownies and potato chips, right? But for the entire two weeks, all you can think about is pizza and brownies and potato chips.

Then the diet is finally over (if you make it). So what do you do? Drive yourself straight to the pizza place and order a large double cheese with a jumbo-sized bag of the saltiest, crispiest, greasiest chips. Then on the way home, you stop at the bakery to buy a box of brownies. And the best part? You don't have to share any of it. You deserve it, after all. You made it two whole weeks without a single bite of your three favorite foods. . . .

So let's just say you don't cave into temptation and you actually do make it through the entire dark woods of denial. You arrive at the edge of the wood with triumph decorating your shoulders. What does your trophy look like? It was supposed to look like your old Barbie doll or that perfect woman on the toothpaste commercial, right? That was the promise you bought into. The pledge of the body you've envisioned for yourself at last finally a reality. And you have made that magic happen with nothing but shear willpower. Why do you do it? Well, of course, it's because once you finally lose that weight, you're going to look better, feel better, date more, buy nicer clothes, and be happy. Life will be just perfect.

If only. . . .

I wouldn't learn until much later that if you begin to move more than you munch, just a little more, almost every day, eat a little less of the foods that I used to call the "devil's gifts" and a lot more of those colorful ones that grow in the ground (you know, God's gifts), you inadvertently begin to find yourself celebrating what's right with the world instead of whining about what's wrong with your body before you even notice you've lost a single pound. And even better: you don't have to push visions of pizza and brownies out of your head, because they never even knocked to get in! That's what I call the win-win approach to reconciliation between food and body image. Seamless. Effortless. Sensible. No-brainer! If I'd only known when I was fourteen what I know now.

Ah, the great game of deprivation endurance.

Deprivation-based diets are the raw material for short-term success stories—and long-term wars with mirrors and food and your thighs and belly. I have the battle-scars to prove it. Making intelligent and sensible choices about food most of the time (notice I said, "most," not "all"), making exercise as routine as brushing your teeth, are the only ways to manage body woes for a lifetime. Well, that's what I thought I'd figured out by the time I hit thirty anyway.

Speaking From Experience: Inspirations to Invite Healing

• **D-I-E-T!**
Diet: (noun) the food eaten in a particular species or culture; (verb) to follow a pattern of restricting food in order to lose weight. . . .

To diet or not to diet—that is the question. Dieting has practically become a national sport. I keep wondering when they're going to enter it into the Olympics! I'm referring to the verb form. You know, to restrict, reduce, control, sometimes even eliminate—food.

Food. What a substance. What a paradox! For so many of us it is simultaneously sustenance and poison. It is fuel, reward, celebration, comfort; then it is venom, torment, anguish. Practically omnipotent, it is capable of transforming a mundane meeting at work into a festive gala, suffocating every last stressful detail of the overflowing inbox of life, filling up emptiness with rich pleasure, and sadness with pure delight . . . . or is it?

We overindulge; we under-indulge. We deprive, restrict, deny and punish ourselves until . . . . we disintegrate.

• Obsession

When we fixate on something—anything—we amplify it. It swells up bigger than an Eiffel Tower-sized Hershey's kiss. What do diets do? They make us fixate on the very thing we are so desperate to stop noticing. They insist images of delectable, mouth-watering, guilty pleasures onto our poor impressionable helpless brains. So what happens? Food becomes larger than life. Or worse—food *becomes* life.

Diets do the opposite of what we want them to do. They tip the scales so far out of balance that we completely lose sight of the fact that there's a whole world of wonderfulness beyond the refrigerator. And then, when life is only about what goes into our mouths, we disappear and we become our bodies. Does that sound like balance to you?

• Good List—Bad List

It seems our species is hardwired to pigeonhole everything in life into distinctly separate slots labeled either "good" or "bad"—strength is good, weakness is bad; laughter is good, tears are bad; wealth is good, poverty is bad; pleasure is good, pain is bad; simplicity is good, difficulty is bad; knowledge is good, ignorance is bad; relationship is good, solitude is bad; clarity is good, confusion is bad.

Exercise is good—calories are bad. Broccoli, salmon, and berries are good—brownies, fried dough, and milk shakes are bad.

What if I told you the only place that "good" and "bad" truly exist is in the mind? What if I were to say it's only about "balance" and "imbalance"?

Here's a short exercise that has helped me to rethink some of my preconceived notions of good versus bad when it comes to food. Perhaps you'll find it helpful too. I target a food that once would have only appeared on the "Bad List" and look for a way it might be permitted onto the "Good List." I consider its merits. "Delicious" is usually the first thing I come up with. Then I take that word "delicious" and I ask myself what could possibly be *wrong* with "delicious"? In and of itself, is it not okay to experience "delicious"? Well, okay then, if "delicious" is not wrong, then what is? Calories? Sugar? Maybe, but it would depend on the conditions. Even calories and sugar have a proper place. Calories are energy. We can't survive without them. Everyone knows that. And what about sugar? As anyone with diabetes knows, sugar can be a superhero in the face of acute low blood glucose. So if sugar has merit, it can't be all bad, right? Drilling down further, I unequivocally isolate the true demon responsible for its position on the Bad List. It always comes down to one thing—imbalance.

Now you try it. What do your answers to these questions tell you about your relationship with food?

2

Verdict: Type 1 Diabetes

The Diagnosis

Let me rewind the calendar a few years. It's 1971. I am in fifth grade. I love school. I love making friends. I love music. I've already composed a few songs of my own and sung them while accompanying myself on guitar. I love walking outside in nature to the soundtrack of bird dialogue and random fanfares of dog barking. Nature's music. I still love playing with dolls now and then too (though I don't admit this to anyone except my friend, Lia).

It's fall—still the beginning of the school year. I have made a few more friends. Making new friends is one of my favorite things to do. Life is fun for ten-year-old me. I'm soaking in all that it has to offer me.

I'm in social studies doing a group project with three of my newest friends. I'm feeling thirsty, so I ask Mrs. Powers if I can get a drink at the bubbler just outside the classroom. She is very kind and gentle.

"Of course," she smiles.

I proceed to the water fountain across the corridor and wait for the water to reach a cool temperature and I lean forward to sip. My mouth and throat are grateful. I begin to gulp and I'm making loud sounds as I swallow. My stomach begins to fill up and expand like a water balloon. My thirst is insatiable.

David Flemming is now behind me, patiently waiting for his turn. "Jeez! You gonna leave any for me?" he finally sighs. "You're hoggin' it all!"

Mild embarrassment halts my consumption and I rejoin my team inside the classroom working on our project. But it's not long before gravity has

9

pulled that voluminous absorption of water from moments ago downward, and I begin to sense an urgent need to use the restroom. I was excused for a second time.

Though I gave very little consideration to that particular episode beyond its annoying and relentless power to cause me typical fifth grade self-consciousness, others identical to it would begin to characterize my first term of fifth grade.

During the holidays that same year, I came down with what was assumed to be the flu. Most of my family was also sick. I remind you, this was 1971 when a commonly used treatment to control vomiting was coke syrup. It was precisely the therapy used on all of us. Though I've never looked at the ingredients listed on the back label of a bottle of coke syrup, I'm pretty certain that it's safe to assume one of the first ingredients is sugar.

Though this mysterious healing potion seemed to calm the ills for my family members, we surmised that I must have contracted a worse case than the rest. I just couldn't stop throwing up. We were all hit pretty hard, but after three or four days, while my family was clearly on the road to recovery, my condition was steadily declining.

My parents had been calling the pediatrician hourly and they diligently followed every instruction. But my body was refusing to respond cooperatively. Now utterly weak, depleted and gaunt, about to step into the tub Mom had just filled for me, I caught the reflection in the bathroom mirror of what used to be my face. There were dark blackish sockets where my eyes used to be. My lips were a dry, scabby brownish color and stuck together when I spoke or swallowed. The inside of my mouth was basted with a film of stickiness. Where was my face? This wasn't me. And what had happened to the rest of my body? You could easily make a ring around my knees with your thumb and middle finger and count every single one of my ribs now clearly visible through my nearly transparent skin.

Straight from the tub, to the pediatrician, to the hospital. Mom's tears. Dad's . . . . *accusations?* Did he think this was Mom's fault? Funny the people who become your scapegoats in the face of fear. So often it's the ones who hold the greatest power to strengthen and support you.

The diagnosis of Juvenile Diabetes must have felt like a death sentence to my parents. I can only say that now, 37 years later . . . . but I couldn't have known it then. At age ten, the world was still all about me.

Type 1 Diabetes is usually diagnosed in children and young adults, and was previously known as juvenile diabetes. In Type 1 Diabetes, the body does not produce insulin.

Two weeks is a mighty long time when you are ten. I spent two weeks in the hospital learning how to inject my thigh with insulin—practicing several times a day on my teddy bear; two weeks learning to test my urine for glucose and ketones; two weeks watching my weight climb from a sickly thirty-five pounds back up to a healthier forty-eight and an even healthier fifty-two; two weeks learning how to measure food into appropriate serving sizes that fit into the Diabetic Food Exchange List categories of meats, breads, fruits, vegetables and fats. Every food had a label, a category, a unit of measure, a value. Two weeks—learning, poking, jabbing, measuring, peeing, counting . . . . and adapting.

Juvenile Diabetes. It would shape the rest of my life in ways I couldn't yet begin to imagine.

Dear God, Thanks for Science

"What did diabetics do in the old days?" I asked my mom one spring afternoon later that same year as we were baking a batch of chocolate chip cookies. I was still getting used to my new set of eating regulations. "Before scientists invented insulin?"

"I'm sure they must have gotten very sick," she answered, "like you did this past Christmas."

"But I wouldn't have gotten better if I didn't have insulin, right?"

"Right. You'll need insulin for the rest of your life."

When you are ten, 'the rest of your life' is as ambiguous as 'maybe' or 'someday' or 'we'll see.' I didn't really mind too much though. Some of the other diabetic kids in the hospital had made such a big deal about the needles, but really, it wasn't so awful.

"What happens if I forget sometime?"

"You'd get sick again, but not as sick as you were on Christmas." How sick would I get, I wondered. My mom must have read the concern in my eyes. She was good at looking inside a child's fear. "I'm sure that we could get you better quickly now that we have insulin right in the house." But I saw straight through her reassuring words. How could she possibly promise that? She couldn't know.

I pushed a spoonful of cookie dough onto the baking sheet and licked off the sweet residue of batter from my index finger. Mom didn't have to say anything. She didn't have to gesture. Her look said it all. It wasn't a scolding look, but more like a firm gentle reminder. Like you'd almost expect to hear, "Don't forget to look both ways next time." She clearly appreciated that it would take me a while to learn my new set of rules, but to me it felt as though I'd just done something as morally wrong as cheating on a math test or stealing a piece of Bazooka bubblegum from the candy bin at the corner five-and-ten shop.

"So what happened to the people who came down with diabetes in the days of Jesus?" Give it to me straight, Mom. Worst-case scenario. What can *really* happen to me if I don't take my shot? I mean like forever? Or maybe just for a long time? "If they didn't have insulin, they wouldn't have ever gotten better, right?"

"No, I don't think they would have been able to."

"So they would have . . . . *died?*"

She hesitated. "I'm sure that's what happened. But there were a lot of diseases back then that weren't treatable. And a lot of people died in those days because science had a lot of growing yet to do."

Science. It was no longer a mere subject in fifth grade where we learned the difference between cumulous and stratus clouds, or neutrons and protons. It was something for which I owed volumes of gratitude. I suppose I owed my life to it.

Bless Me Father, for I Have Just Eaten Chocolate Pudding

One of the most radical diets I ever tried was one I made up myself when I was fourteen. It amounted to precisely six hundred calories a day—not a single calorie more. I took the task of designing the diet quite seriously, studiously researching and computing the caloric values of any food that would become part of the overall plan. The exactness of that diet is still etched in my brain. . . .

Breakfast:
one scrambled egg (NO oil)
half a grapefruit

Lunch:
one can of tuna (dry—NO mayo)
on top of iceberg lettuce
drizzled with vinegar and lemon juice

Dinner:
exactly two ounces of fish or chicken (NO toppings, marinades or frills)
served with cucumber slices

NO snacks. NO exceptions. NO matter what! (My self-designed "NO" diet.)

I was at that age when some girls begin gaining adolescent body fat around the middle, around the same time as The Green Dress—not really enough to make me look like a teenage waddle or anything, but just enough for the mirror to start scolding and shaming me. I was about five feet tall at the time and weighed in at around ninety pounds. I detested the new pot-belly look I'd recently begun to sport and I decided to take matters into my own hands and aggressively attempted to reclaim my ten-year-old body.

I think it was around the fourth or fifth day of rigidly abiding by the rules of that made-up diet when I felt all sensation leave my fingertips. Lightheaded and limp, I was scared. I remember thinking that God might be punishing me for not sticking to the diabetic diet I was supposed to be following.

My hands continued to tingle with numbness as I desperately and violently tore open the refrigerator and urgently devoured anything that looked the remotest bit forbidden to my ravenous, diabetic-caged self. Ah, freedom at last! I'd removed the handcuffs of both diabetes and self-imposed starvation in a single act. I had escaped Diabetic Prison!

I came across a large bowl of chocolate pudding and in that moment all the forbidden fruits from the Garden of Eden (or the Garden of EATING!) were mine. I remember taking a spoon straight to the refrigerator and repeatedly dipping it into that bowl. I ate, and ate, and ate, and ate—until the bowl had nothing left to offer me.

And in less than an instant, frenzied lust for sweet forbidden chocolate turned the ugly corner of shame and guilt. What had I done? All the calories. All the sugar. All the regret. There was no turning back. It wasn't possible to now *un-eat* what I had just moments ago practically inhaled like a human vacuum cleaner. My choices were limited: I could take some extra insulin to cover my crimes of passion and risk another face-off with the bathroom-scale-bully; or I could walk deeper into the familiar dark woods that stood before me, that place where I'd already dared to travel before, that place where the lifelessness of *diabetic ketoacidosis* brutally purges all your "sins."

I skipped my insulin that night. It was my penance.

The next day I lay in my hospital bed with five intravenous tubes connecting the insides of my arms, ankles, and neck to the stark walls of that room. There was not a single ounce of energy left in me. My mouth was drier than Arizona sand. My stomach felt as though it had expelled every morsel of food I had ever eaten. The muscles along my torso felt bruised from endless violent heaving; my insides now entirely evacuated. The combination of this torturous diet and the resulting chocolate pudding binge had and cost me two collapsed lungs and nearly ten pounds of weight loss, consisting not of fat, mind you, but primarily of essential body fluids.

13

I hated the person lying in that hospital bed. Hated her and the enormity of her weakness; hated her for caving in to the temptation of chocolate pudding; for deliberately breaking all the rules of diabetic-hood; for all of her broken promises. And all the hate for that fourteen-year-old girl lying helpless in a hospital bed, vehemently found its channel through the cruel and unforgiving judge inside.

Shame was spilling out of me now. My insides felt as toxic as a pungent sewer. But I deserved it. I had done it to myself.

Speaking From Experience: Inspirations to Invite Healing

• Freedom and Responsibility

Human beings are the only living organisms on the planet both blessed and burdened with free will. Freedom—the glorious ability to choose our own actions, thoughts, beliefs, feelings. But with freedom comes implicit responsibility. We are accountable to make the right choice. When we believe we have chosen rightly, it is freeing. It is the responsibility of freedom and the freedom of responsibility. Neither exists apart from the other.

When it comes to food, free will can sometimes feel more like a curse than a privilege, especially immersed in a culture abundant with super-sized indulgences that bombard us at every corner. With such easy, unobstructed access to irresponsible choices everyday, we find we must call upon the strength of the mind in order to drive our choosing in the right direction. And so we flex the almighty willpower muscle.

How do we define willpower? Determination? Discipline? Drive? Self-control? Where does it come from? How can we develop more of it? Willpower is an inner strength of the mind that empowers us to do the "right" thing—or what we *perceive* to be the "right" thing—despite the difficulties involved. And when we nail that, we feel amazing, right?

• Flexing the Willpower Muscle

I'd like to ask you, do you believe willpower is supposed to be stronger than authentic hunger? If hunger is nature's signal that the body is in immediate need of fuel for optimum anatomical functioning, then why would we want to overpower that signal? To compromise anatomical functioning couldn't possibly ever be a worthy objective, so how could we believe that telling our appetite to shut up is a good thing? Do we not understand that it "speaks" with good reason?

I'm not talking about the kind of appetite that is rooted in boredom, loneliness, overtiredness, sadness, failure, or stress. I promise you—that kind of hunger will never be truly satisfied with food. No, I'm talking about the kind of hunger that stomps its foot and "yells" at you because you've eaten nothing but a few celery stalks for the past eight hours. *That* kind of hunger needs to be heard. So listen to it—kindly, patiently. If you are genuinely hungry, your body needs fuel, so for the love of God, *EAT!*

• Filling the Space with Value

Why not start with something colorful (and I don't mean jelly beans). Try something that comes straight from the earth without taking several detours on its journey to your lips—in short, not that processed stuff that only pretends to be food. Grab a handful of bright red juicy strawberries direct from the local farmer's market to your mouth. Or try a different color—green, maybe. Some crisp sugar snap peas or a ripe juicy kiwi. Now, how about a few of those vibrant orange sweet potato wedges? Go ahead. Let that rainbow explode in your mouth and paint the inside of your stomach! Once you've eaten a rainbow, let's do some texture—crunchy almonds, velvety yogurt, chewy whole grain bread.

Now, I challenge you to find a little space inside that chamber of nourishment for one tiny innocent little brownie or harmless spoonful of chocolate pudding. What? You no longer want it? Need I say more?

3

When Body Image and Diabetes Collide

Music, Drama, and Donuts

1979 was a big year. In June, I graduated from high school. In July, my parents separated. In August, I moved into the city to live with my aunt Joan (my favorite cook in the world) so that I could commute to Boston Conservatory of Music. In September, I began my freshman year. Music had been everything to me in high school and acceptance to the conservatory represented validation and renewal. A fresh start. A clean slate. (I was always searching for the next clean slate.)

Freshman orientation was equally overwhelming and electrifying. I was introduced to all kinds of unique characters that day—musicians, professors, drama coaches, vocal instructors, classmates, and a brand new world of eclectic and, in some instances, effeminate men. I sat through assemblies, bought supplies, followed tours of Boston, and designed my schedule. I was a Musical Theater major, so my classes covered the entire spectrum of music and drama. There would be voice lessons twice a week, three-hour drama classes on Wednesday afternoons, music theory on Fridays, public speaking on Tuesdays, playwright history on Mondays, and all kinds of dance classes—ballet, tap, jazz, modern—for two to four hours every day—including Saturday mornings.

Two to four hours a day—of *dancing*. I'd never have to diet again! Heck, a schedule saturated with this level of inherent calorie burning, might actually permit me to even eat some of my aunt Joan's mouth-watering recipes and still lose weight!

By the end of the first week, the bathroom scale in my aunt Joan's apartment spoke poetry to my ears. It was more magical than every particle of Tinkerbelle's fairy dust, more magical than Tinkerbelle herself. I had lost five pounds without skipping a single meal or a single shot all week. I even had a few low blood sugars that needed to be treated with candy—straight up. At this rate, I could conjure up any body I wanted for my own, and it would be mine. This was extreme euphoria. No doubt, the single solution to all my diet woes of high school.

The next week, I knew it was time for me to find a part-time job so that I would be able to afford a second semester at the conservatory. I walked along Central Street in West Roxbury and submitted applications at a few of the jewelry shops and boutiques. When I had exhausted all possibilities there, I proceeded to Roslindale Square. The shops were less appealing, but it was that much closer to my subway stop so I figured I'd give it a whirl. The two Greek brothers who owned the Dunkin' Donuts on the corner were eager to hire me. When can I start? What shifts am I available? Can I work full-time on Sundays?

I started on the late shift, 7:00 pm–1:00 am, beginning the following Friday night. My uniform was a bright pink baseball-type hat, a pink, orange and white button down blouse, and a beige bibbed apron, all with the Dunkin' Donuts logo. I kind of liked what I looked like wearing it (though it's likely I would have approved of any new look after losing eight pounds in two weeks).

I worked hard at the conservatory during the day and moonlighted at Dunkin' Donuts at night. And I continued to steadily and reliably lose weight, though my rate was beginning to slow down to about a pound a week.

1979 was a big year. A *very* big year. In October, my parents divorced. I had just closed a one-act play in which I had been awarded a leading role. I was the only freshman in the cast and I felt honored and privileged (okay, maybe even a little "diva"). But the fatigue of moonlighting at Dunkin' Donuts, the wear and tear of ten hours of grueling sweat-spilling dance lessons a week, the inner unrest of emotional digging during drama classes, and the raw open wounds of a newly broken family-life, were upstaging my enthusiasm for this new world.

And I found consolation in a box of donuts. One dozen of the most alluring, seductive, mouth-watering, drool-producing unique varieties of that corner donut shop in Roslindale Square.

It was 1:00 am. My shift was over. I pretended I was going to a brunch back home the following morning and I was in charge of bringing a dozen donuts. It seemed a harmless fabrication. How could I possibly confess that this box was really intended for none other than its buyer? And it contained every single evil temptation that had tormented me since I first worked there.

I drove out of Roslindale Square and pulled into the empty parking lot at St. Theresa's Church in West Roxbury. I opened the pink and orange cardboard box and feasted my eyes on this package of sinfulness. I pulled out a Bavarian cream. I'd never before tasted one of these and for the past two months it had been calling out to me louder than any other. I took a single bite. Every tooth was now lavishly caressed by the sweet texture of flaky bliss. Smooth vanilla flooded my mouth with creamy pleasure. I savored every bite of that first donut. And then, I approached my second, a toasted coconut—crunchy bits of praline-like morsels surrounding a doughy ring of heaven. By the third, the magnetic pull of that box of temptation was beginning to weaken. I panicked. This was to be a one-time-only event. What if I didn't have the stamina for all of these donuts? This was my one and only chance to cover all bases, to sample every donut that had been torturing me with its promise of forbidden delicious ecstasy these past months.

Each of these diabetic criminals had just as much right to be relished by me as the one beside it. So in an effort to elongate pleasure and maximize endurance, I changed my approach. A single bite. Move on to the next. And the next. And the next . . . . each bite taking up more room in the limited space inside my stomach. And as that limited space filled, pleasure diminished proportionally.

My aunt Joan knew little about my disease. She wouldn't have the faintest idea that my incessant throwing up that night had anything to do with some secret donut binge and its resulting sugar high. She wouldn't suspect a thing. And she wouldn't even learn I was sick until the next morning when I would say, "I must have caught some lousy stomach bug."

Investigating the reasons for your sugar binges and addressing the reasons for them, might help you enjoy sweets in moderation. Denying oneself all sweets can become a common binge motivator.

1979. My world had changed much too suddenly. I was lost in a foreign world of drama disguised as reality, reality disguised as drama, culture shock of gay artsy men to which I'd never before been exposed, and acute family injury. I left Boston Conservatory at the end of October and moved back home. It had been a big year.

Torments of a Large Extra Cheese

It was too late in the year for me to restart my freshman year at another college so I spent the rest of that school year adjusting to divorce and becoming a new and improved me. I would work hard—two jobs—so that I would have plenty of money to afford both college and a complete new wardrobe for my next attempt at the freshman experience. I would improve my mind by reading all the classics I missed in high school and borrowing my younger, brainier (not to mention prettier and skinnier) sister's word-lists from Advanced English III in order to enhance my vocabulary. And I would improve my body by losing ten or even twenty pounds. It was possible. I had a whole year to become the person I wanted to be and start all over again.

I returned to my old high school part-time job at the local pizza place and made it my full-time job for the rest of that year. I also took on an additional job at Cumberland Farms next door so that I could toggle back and forth between the two—lunchtime sub-maker, afternoon cashier, and dinnertime pizza-cutter. Fifty to seventy hours a week. They were long hours without many breaks. And they were long hours to stare down temptation.

But I was determined to become a better me, so I spent a lot of effort strengthening my immunity to pizza—numbing my sense of smell to the savory aroma of basil and tomato, and my sense of sight to the irresistible vision of warm, gooey, bubbly cheese sliding off soft doughy pizza crust. I had grown up in a love affair with pizza, but it had become one of those foods from the self-constructed list of no-no's that was now part of my internal wiring.

It was a lonely time. Craving both comfort and companionship, I was disappearing into a world that used to belong to me. My friends were away at college. My siblings were still in school. My parents were estranged. On occasion, I might experience a tiny bit of respite from all of this isolation through the charitable heart of my sister Therese when, in addition to loaning me her vocabulary lists, she also loaned me her circle of friends, inviting me along (almost as if *I* were the younger sibling). But for the most part, I felt alone with my books, my vocabulary lists—and my temptations.

The busy dinner hours began to dwindle down to a few random customers as my shift was ending one night. There was a large extra cheese pizza that had been awaiting its pickup for over two hours when it was time for me to leave. Panos, the owner, asked me if I'd like to take it home? I accepted politely and began my two-mile walk toward Spring Street.

When you're walking through the park alone at dusk and your only companion is the sweet smell of tomato sauce and mozzarella, when loneliness prevails and comfort eludes you, there is nothing quite as soothing as a large extra cheese pizza. I found a wooden bench and opened the box, the imprisoned sweet spicy fragrance escaping in a single wave. The two-hour-old pizza was still just as alluring to me as it had been in its steamy infancy. I slid out a slice and took a bite. What's the big deal, I thought? It's just one piece of innocent *pizza*—not a mortal sin! Plenty of thin people eat pizza all the time and don't gain weight. But when you've yearned for reward and comfort and satisfaction and friendship for so long and suddenly pleasure reaches that deep inside of you, one piece is not enough.

From one piece to the entire pizza. And then the familiar heap of solid mass in my stomach. It was heavier than gravity itself this time. And it was relentless. I still had another mile to walk before I could barf in my own 'barf'-room. I arose from the park bench and attempted to take my first step. This was going to be a long arduous mile home. A second step . . . . then a third and a fourth. My throat contracted. My tongue pushed down . . . . then I gagged. Impossible. How was I to get my hundred-pound body, now sad-dled with weighty clumps of greasy, tomatoey, mozzarella and thick bready pizza crust from this park to 146 Spring Street? It wasn't going to happen. I groaned. I cried. I crawled. What an odd vision that must have been—a fully-grown young woman crawling in the park! But concern with appearances had no place in my actions now. Occasionally, I tried to walk again . . . . slowly. I rested against a tree. I stayed there for ten minutes or so. I slid down the side of that tree and leaned my head against its trunk. And I slipped away from consciousness. . . .

I'm not sure how long I slept, but when I awoke, I ran to the metal trash barrel beside the seesaw. I had no choice at that point. That pizza was racing full speed through my throat toward the exit door of my mouth . . . . and it spilled straight into that trash barrel.

Please God, I begged. Please make me stop doing this.

There was no such thing as a cell phone then, so I couldn't let Mom know I was okay. And I *was* okay—now that my stomach had pushed out all of that evil. I was empty again. Another clean slate. I could walk again. It was dark, but I knew Mom wouldn't ask for an explanation. Now practically a self-supporting member of our broken household, I was the least of her concerns. There were still five younger sisters and brothers for her to parent all alone.

The Perfect Paradigm

I suppose on some level, I had become aware of my bulimia by the time I entered Stonehill College the following September (though I hadn't yet known it actually had a name). Once again, I was the freshman rookie, but there was no déjà vu here. Stonehill College and Boston Conservatory were polar opposites, practically erected on different planets. The multi-cultural backdrop of Boston's cello-hauling Vivaldi-wannabe's, Harvard pre-meds, Fenway Park, and city smog versus countryside sprawling landscapes with academic buildings clustered into neighborhood-like communities, meticulously manicured gardens surrounding Madonna statues, and an abundant population of eligible Catholic athletes with crew cuts and Izod rugby shirts. New scenery. New major. New home. New life. New me. It was time to reinvent myself. Time to put aside foolish whims of Broadway and chorus lines and begin to drink up visions of perfect Catholic weddings, white picket fences and family cookouts.

Freshmen year had its ups and downs, both on and off the scale. My dorm wing was a self-made family of freshman girls. And like good "sisters," we supported each other in our goal to escape the "Freshman Fifteen." We dieted together, binged together, partied together, and dieted again. . . . together.

By the end of my freshman year, I had gotten very chummy with a sweet, bright, and adorable biology major. She was short—like me. She was blonde—*not* like me, but like the skinny "me" of my imagination (having fully embraced the miracle of Sun-In during my high school years). Her eyes lit up when dinner conversation zeroed in on diet woes—like me. And she was thin. *Very* thin. I emulated her.

Together we dieted. We ran. We obsessed. We commiserated over fat and triumphed over thin. We went on the four-day 9-a-day Diet. . . .

Day one—9 boiled eggs. Nothing else.
Day two—9 bananas. Nothing else.
Day three—9 hot dogs. Nothing else.
Day four—3 eggs, 3 bananas, 3 hot dogs. Nothing else.

We supported each other on the campus-wide two-week Scarsdale Diet. I'd finally met my match. I could fixate on losing weight completely jeer-free. I indulged in this rare opportunity to talk "diet" as much as I wanted, though I must admit, I didn't understand *her* obsession a single bit. She was already perfect.

I suppose what really drew me to my Stonehill friend was that she made me feel like I wasn't the only one who thought about food all the time. Meeting her gave me permission to be me. I stopped feeling so alone with myself; stopped feeling like the loser I'd taken myself to be. *She* wasn't a loser after all, so how could I be if we had so much in common? I was in awe of her. And after awhile, I became eager to learn how she was able to eat so much, and weigh so little.

And it would be this intelligent, adorable, perfect, skinny new friend of mine that would unknowingly teach me about the way of non-diabetic purging—self-induced vomiting.

By the end of my sophomore year, my friend was spending a lot of time at the campus mental health center. It was the first time I'd ever heard the word, anorexia. But I didn't really need to hear the word. I'd already known the illness.

Though I recognized that I shared my friend's unhealthy relationship with food, I decided that I couldn't possibly have the same "disease" she had. I wasn't skinny enough to be anorexic. There was no name for my psychosis. I was just emotionally malformed and neurotic. A pathological loser after all. From where I stood, despite her agonizing relationship with food, deep down I felt envious of her anorexia. At least it made her thin. Uncontrollably perhaps, painfully perhaps, but thin just the same. In my corner of the world, thin was still life's remedy for all discontent. Maybe by being her friend, I could "learn" to become anorexic too. Maybe I could even *catch* her anorexia. If I could catch it, I wouldn't even *want* to eat anymore. I wouldn't have to wrestle with all the temptations that continued to torture me day after day, year after year. And I would never again be compelled to drive my blood sugar to that crippling high that stripped any semblance of aliveness from my body and my spirit. I could eat what I wanted—which would be nothing, if I could achieve anorexia—and just live for a change.

It would take years for me to attempt my friend's purging technique, the finger-down-the-throat trick. It wasn't pleasant. But worse, it wasn't nearly as productive as I'd expected it to be. "After all I ate . . . . and *this* is all that comes up!" I remember being appalled at the scant amount of regurgitated food in the toilet bowl. I tried it a few more times however, and I did get better at it, but I still found my purging method much more productive. With insulin omission, I could not only erase a just-gone-by binge, I could often even surpass it. Though I never stopped dreading the debilitating sickness after an episode, I decided that it was a comparatively small price to pay in proportion to such an enormous drop on the scale. In the end, I concluded that between my friend and me, I was actually the one who had this purging thing much easier.

I became increasingly familiar with my boundaries for tolerating the unbearable ills of self-induced *diabetic ketoacidosis* and pushed it to the edge often. My "*ketoacidosis* threshold," I called it. I grew masterful at hiding my secret physical and psychological powerlessness behind feigned optimism and contrived joviality. And from that place of pretend happy-go-lucky, I created a full circle of collegiate wealth, including academics, drama club, music ministry, and an explosive social life (much better than the one I longed for in high school). But privately stuck in a world of broken love and self-loathing, I continued cycles of bingeing for my emotional highs, and omitted insulin for my butt-and-thigh lows.

Alcoholics may be well aware of the risks of taking that first sip; drug abusers may be aware of the dangers of overdosing; and I was *aware* of the irreparable and even life-threatening damage that all this blood sugar foul-play threatened to cause my heart, kidneys, eyes, nerves—heck, the whole body! But it didn't stop me. I was addicted to a partnership of polar opposites—the pleasure of eating and the high of starvation.

At the end of my senior year, following a series of broken melodramas, I met Russ. We fell in love and married in 1986. The slate was once again wiped clean for the next reinvention of me.

Speaking From Experience: Inspirations to Invite Healing

• **The Woman in the Mirror**
The Tibetans have a saying: "One who looks not with compassion sees not what the eyes of compassion see."

Are you one of the millions who look in the mirror and see nothing but flaws?

Do you plaster makeup on your face to cover up a dark freckle or draw attention away from your nose? Maybe you belt a long blouse to create the illusion of a thinner waist, or jam your toes into ultra pointy high-heeled pumps trying to make your legs look long enough to wrap around Gillette Stadium. Do these strategies sound even a little familiar? I'm not suggesting it's damaging or meaningless to pay attention to such things, but let's be clear about where their authentic value lies.

• **The Difference Between Artistry and Beauty**
Imagine a favorite place that brings you back to the blithe days of early childhood. What would a painting of this intimately special place look like? No matter how talented the artist might be, could his painting of your favorite place ever begin to approach the reality

that's still alive in your memory? Which is more alive—the painting, or the memory?

Makeup and fashion are much like the painting—art in their own right, but hardly suitable rivals for *real*.

So what will it be—the innovation of today's newest cosmetics and trendy apparel or the person inside them; a colorful watercolor landscape on a piece of flat one-dimensional canvas or that sacred space in your mind where childhood lives forever; the size, shape, and color of some image in the mirror . . . . or the pure essence of self that fills up every square inch of your very own skin? By mistaking any of these for the other, my fear is that we may inadvertently cast shadows on the most authentic beauty of all.

• **Reflect**

If you answered yes to my very first question, "Are you one of the millions who look in the mirror and see nothing but flaws?" think about the following:

1. times when you felt loved, even though you didn't look "perfect"
2. people you love who don't look "perfect"
3. "perfect"-looking people who act so awful they appear ugly

Now look in the mirror. Who do you see?

BROKEN

4

Somewhere Between Extremes and Balance

The Edge

Russ entered my world with a complete resume of credentials qualifying him to become the husband of a woman with diabetes. As a teenager he had worked as a night supervisor at Carroll Center for the Blind where the majority of patients were so afflicted due to poorly controlled diabetes. He had all the basics of diabetes down pat well before life happened to put us together. The only thing he knew of my obsession with my weight, however, was that, like many women my age, I aimed to push it closer to the left side of the number line. He was oblivious to the notion that these two conditions were so closely related.

I saw marriage as another beginning, a true reason to change. I was motivated and determined to live life from this point forward as "normal" married couples live—children, a nice home, holiday gatherings with family, summer vacations, and maybe even a white picket fence. Sound cliché? Truth is, my vision of married life at that juncture *was* a cliché. Or maybe it was simply that I romanticized its power to release me from a very private hell.

For several months before my wedding, I followed the Diet Workshop plan I had borrowed from my sister-in-law-to-be. Like so many of the chronic dieters I'd already shared space with during my lifetime, she was ostensibly well versed on the topic of dieting. She was a true advocate of this particular one and had extolled the virtues of it often. Eager to begin a less radical approach to becoming thin for the I-do's of life's next chapter, I enthusiastically hopped on board. Coincidentally, the Diet Workshop plan was nearly identical to The Diabetic Exchange List I had been taught to follow when I was first diagnosed with diabetes, so it's not surprising that my blood sugars inadvertently improved.

I was caught off guard by the many delightfully unexpected consequences of my improving blood sugar management. It was easier to get up in the morning. I felt energized and vibrant. Finding motivation for exercise no longer felt like an impossible scavenger hunt. I was sleeping better with fewer midnight trips to the bathroom. Weight loss, though less immediate, was becoming predictable and consistent. Amazingly, for the first time since viewing my body in that notorious green dress, it was also beginning to feel less urgent. My blood sugar, my general disposition, my body weight, and life on the whole were growing even-tempered and serene. Relaxed, unthreatening, effortless—even *fun*. This must be what it feels like not to have diabetes, I remember thinking. I hadn't felt this "normal" since I was eight. Living with this kind of internal environment was like taking some sort of Diabetic Prozac!

For Type 1 Diabetics, purposeful blood sugar control walks a fine line between healthy management and irrepressible obsession. Being a "good diabetic" and living with an eating disorder share a lot of common ground. Both require diligent attention to food and to body weight. Perpetual calculation and accuracy are imperative, as both of these demand accountability for every morsel of food that passes your lips. And just to make matters more confusing, candy is forbidden in one moment and in the next it becomes a life-saving medicine.

As I've explained, eating too much sugar without sufficient insulin can cause a diabetic's blood sugar to climb to potentially dangerous, even fatal levels. But not eating *enough* can be equally risky, and sometimes even more so. It can cause blood sugar levels to plummet to acutely life-threatening concentrations. These are the moments when candy, or any form of sugar, is transformed from an outlawed no-no, to a vitally essential drug.

The five packs of Life Savers® that had now taken up permanent residence at the bottom of my Liz Claiborne bag were medically necessary fixtures, the most critical instruments of a traveling first aid kit—portable, out of sight, and highly effective when under fire of low blood sugar. And at only eight calories each, they could hardly impede whatever weight loss strategy happened to be the mission of the hour—unless for some unknown reason low blood sugar happened to decide to incessantly attack regularly throughout the course of an entire day. A reading of 41 in the middle of a workday was really no major barrier to weight loss. The additional 56 calories from seven lifesavers was miniscule enough to offset the following day during my workout. But seven times in the same day? That required almost 400 unplanned calories—more than an entire meal!

Good blood sugar control may well have felt like Diabetic Prozac but the tightrope upon which it required me to balance was thin, and it was mighty difficult in this land of diabetic happy-hood to keep from falling into the claws of the ominous low.

Blood sugar lows can result in:
- hunger
- shakiness
- sweating
- dizziness
- sleepiness
- confusion
- anxiety
- weakness
- difficulty speaking

I had become so diligent about calorie restriction that I had begun to ignore the signs of low blood sugar in favor of preventing additional sugar and calorie consumption. Then I stopped noticing them altogether. They even disappeared entirely for a time. On a few occasions during the first few months of our marriage, I experienced seizures from these lows. These occasions were frightening to my new husband and he bought me my very first blood glucose meter. We had planned on children in our future and we both appreciated the value of proactively hauling my disease into the safe zone.

With Russ's supportive gentle nudging (okay, maybe it was more like a firm push), I admitted myself to Joslin Clinic Teaching Unit for a two-week stay. There, I would re-educate myself about my disease and, for the very first time in my twenty-five year life, begin to transform my unhealthy ways and stabilize my blood sugars.

The zone of perfection was 80-120. That was my target, but hardly ever my reality. While I wasn't expected to fall in that range each and every time, *"periodically-to-frequently"* would have been a welcome change. Heck, with my history, I'd even settle for *sporadically*. If I based my insulin adjustments on these numbers, perhaps I might come closer to the ideal more regularly before working on becoming pregnant.

For months after my stay in Joslin Clinic, my history with weight obsession morphed into a fixation with blood sugar control. I tested my levels hourly and recorded every single result. At the close of each day, I would sit and analyze the data in an attempt to extrapolate all relevant information that promised to improve my control for the following day. I received a very satisfying reward too. My A1C, the result of a blood test that evaluates your past three-month blood sugar average, was 6.2 (the non-diabetic range was under 5.4). For someone with Type 1 Diabetes, this was perfect. Heck, *I* was perfect in this moment. I felt like I had just received an A+ on the diabetic report card! My self-worth was still based on a number, but at least it wasn't the one on the bathroom scale.

My newly acquired preoccupation with blood sugar control felt oddly familiar to me. It was the same obsession wearing a new outfit. But there was one principle difference between blood sugar obsession and weight loss obsession. Unlike weight loss obsession, this new bee had flown into my bonnet fully clad as a *healthy* objective. And it *was* healthy—for a while.

If you are walking along the edge of a cliff and a strong wind stirs your balance, you're likely to run away from that edge to keep from falling off. At what point do diligence and commitment become the neurotic and self-destructive pursuit of impossible perfection? I have walked this cliff many times. It is hard not to fall off. And when my balance wavers and fear of falling panics me, I have run frightfully from that edge. But life's wisdom is presented to us in many packages and it *is* possible to begin learning—one step at a time—how to walk along the edge without falling off. I was still learning to walk. And it was very hard to balance.

Magic

Picture this: After spending a lifetime dreaming up visions of a human Barbie doll as your personal idol, you wake up one day and hop on the scale you've been hiding underneath your bed for months. Ninety-two, it reads.

You suddenly realize that—at least in the "important" ways (the tiny waist, the pencil-thin legs, practically invisible buttocks)—you're beginning to approach that "some-day vision" that has existed in your head since you began eighth grade. The dream you had once given up for dead is actually starting to look like it might be possible after all.

Then, Friday night at the cocktail party after work, once you finish your first glass of Merlot, you start to feel almost beautiful. The denim fabric of your size 0 jeans is feeling baggy around your thighs and waistline, the bones of your ribcage seem to have very little anatomical matter covering them besides a thin layer of skin, and while the black suede shoes with four-inch heels are beginning you make your feet ache, it's well worth the extra length they give your legs.

The next morning, you awake with a pounding headache and crippling clump of regret anchoring you to the bed. You suddenly recall all the hors d'oeuvres you inhaled last night, once the second glass of Merlot had finally paralyzed your stubborn willpower—the pumpernickel cubes and artichoke dip, the cheesy potato skins, the hummus and pita chips.

Now imagine you have access to this amazing magic: an illness that lets you eat everything you could possibly ever want and still lose even more weight—the more you eat, the more you lose. Stacks of pancakes and French toast drenched in maple syrup for breakfast; grilled paninis with peanut butter, fluff and partially melted chocolate chips for lunch; heaps of buttery pasta and warm crusty white bread for dinner; even a mammoth slice of praline pecan cheesecake with gooey caramel drizzle for dessert! Heck, you might even decide to eat the entire pie! Why not? This miraculous disease you have will make you drop five or maybe even ten pounds by tomorrow morning—as long as you eat everything in sight and then skip your insulin.

Of course, there are a few hitches: you'll be utterly exhausted, you won't be able to focus on anything, you might lose some of your hair, your fingertips will tingle and then go numb, and there's this putrid taste in your mouth that no amount of toothpaste or mouthwash is able to exterminate. Keep going with this miracle diet and you'll probably go blind someday, lose your feet, or die of kidney failure or a sudden heart attack. But in the meantime, you've been able to eat as many Snickers® bars and M&Ms® as you wanted and still watch the pounds just melt away.

Now I ask you honestly, if you had access to that kind of magic, what would *you* do with it?

Baby Steps

Everything we do in life is either a step toward or a step away from balance. *Everything.* The direction we're headed depends entirely on where we are before we move. If I'm already in balance, then whatever I do will move me away from balance. If I am out of balance, then whatever I do will either move me closer to balance or further away from it, depending on what I choose to do.

Late in the eighties, I decided to take on my war with food, disease, and body image full force. Game on! I joined a clinical study on the benefits of exercise on diabetics. A year later, I became a fitness instructor. Intense physical activity became the healthy substitute for those ugly sugar highs on the relentless, unchanging battlefield of weight loss. I began to recognize my grueling workouts as the sole victor in my epic crusade against The Fat Zone.

There is no doubt in my mind that I chose to enter the fitness profession because, on some level, I believed that choosing this line of work would keep me thin. I could rationalize to myself that thinness was practically a vocational requisite rather than a measure of personal worth or a vanity wish. No longer my choice—my responsibility. Seeing physical exercise as a job requirement rather than as a personal choice would force my hand. It was a desperate insurance policy to give me the upper hand in my private war.

The battlefield of body image was personal, but I had convinced myself that there was a higher calling to fitness. I'd begun to believe that with my personal history in this war, I could make a difference in the way that we look at ourselves. I suppose that was a bit sanctimonious of me, and was perhaps driven by my hunger for self-importance at the time. Today I know the singular motive: I needed to change the way I looked at *myself.* In the beginning anyway, it was only about me, no matter what higher cause I pretended to stand for. It wouldn't be until decades later, after taking the hard journey inside and peeling away layers of body-obsession to expose the treasure hidden at the core of it all, that the gravitational pull to the world of fitness would be transformed into a truer, deeper purpose.

For the first few years of my work in fitness, I focused on "outer" fitness (you know, the stuff you can actually *see*—like six-pack abs, chiseled shoulders, toned glutes and thighs). Somewhere in there, my understanding of fitness began to evolve and recruit the inner goings-on of the human anatomy. I taught group exercise classes at local health clubs and simultaneously worked my way up my personal fitness ladder. I gradually began to put aside my single-minded focus on weight loss in favor of other fitness goals like muscle strength, endurance and heart health. Though I must confess, I never stopped embracing the perks of my career (such as finally qualifying for the size zero marathon!). I approached food as though it were no longer one of life's pleasures to be consumed (or denied), but rather a medicine to be ingested with precision, based purely on biological requirements. I worked my brain and my body industriously to become the wisest fittest new me possible. I built a portfolio of specialty fitness, nutrition, and wellness certifications and integrated my personal knowledge of this exciting subject matter into every thread of my lifestyle. Life in *The Fit Lane* may not have awarded me the same instant gratification of steep drops of poundage generated by nasty sugar highs, but it was more dependable and productive. And ultimately, it was much longer lasting.

I began to reawaken to some of the inedible pleasures of life, pleasures independent of calorie expenditure values—friendship, music, fresh air, sunshine, shopping, social life, (okay, sex too). I was beginning to taste balance. Once you know that taste, there isn't a single food on God's earth that tastes good enough to give that up.

Funny thing about balance though. It has a way of unexpectedly shifting on you.

Rollercoaster Ride

Life gives us boundaries everywhere. They define our living space. They define our breathing room. Sometimes we push them, just a little, and we soar. Other times we plummet.

The margin for diabetic harmony is narrow. Anything between 80ml/dl and 120ml/dl feels simply delightful. 160ml/dl is about as far as you can stray from normal before "simply delightful" becomes a distant memory. But when the numbers begin to creep up past 250, you begin to feel thirsty and groggy. Once you skyrocket past 400, the intrusion of nausea is unmistakable. The thirst has now invaded every living molecule inside you and releases something that feels like sticky pastiness inside your mouth and eyes. You start to feel shamefully filthy and grungy, as if you hadn't showered for weeks or even months. Then, just when you thought you couldn't feel any worse, life throws in a heaping dose of intense fatigue partnered with a headache the size of Texas! And if the numbers continue to climb? Well it's that familiar debilitation all over again. You may as well just erase the day. There is nothing worthwhile that will come of it from this place. Funny thing though: The whole time this is happening to you, you know you have the power to fix it. All you have to do is draw up some insulin and injected into your leg or your belly. There's only one problem: You'll probably gain weight if you do.

It is very fragile, this diabetic balance. Sometimes you own account-ability of your misery by way of your own actions (a few unplanned harm-less strawberries, a second glass of milk, a couple of extra innocent handfuls of popcorn, a few knife-licks as you cut the brownies you just baked for the party), but often, high blood sugar has a mind of its own, irrationally attack-ing you from behind without notice or provocation. . . . but you still think, it must be my fault. Maybe I ate something without counting it, or maybe I just underestimated or lost track of what I *did* eat.

Low blood sugar has the same sort of multiple personality disorder, a regu-lar Dr. Jekyll and Mr. Hyde. It can be ever so polite, waiting for its "invitation" in the form of a delayed meal or an extra long run; or it can crash your party, rudely knocking you down as it enters. 59. . . 42. . . 26! When it shows up, panic and weakness unite to produce a violently ravenous hunger that is untamable.

Urgency grows. Trembling with sweat that comes from nowhere, turning icy cold as it exits the pores of your skin. Convulsion generates from your center. Until you find yourself standing in front of the candy drawer in the kitchen. Ah, relief is moments away. Candy-corns. You count them. Fifteen. They are medicine in this moment, not a forbidden treat. You con-sume them deliberately. You know in your head that fifteen is the proper dose. You've already scrutinized the nutrition information panel on the side of the bag and done the math well before this moment. But the hunger is now eating your insides.

Panic and weakness continue to grow. They begin to dominate you and overpower your free will. Your body and your mind are now at war. Your body's unrelenting hunger tells your mind that food is immediately critical for its survival. But your mind knows the fifteen candy corns will take effect soon and tame the inner beast. Sometimes the mind is strong enough to overcome the body's hunger, but not always.

The war ends, just moments later. No matter who wins, the rational mind or the uncontrollable hunger of the body, an overwhelming sleepiness smothers the energy you used to know only minutes ago. You are cold, shivering uncontrollably—unable to find warmth anywhere. The coldness seems to come from within. And it won't go away.

It is a long way from here to diabetic calm. If the mind—or the *will*—has been this war's victor, you sleep for a while and simply awake with a headache. But if the body's unyielding hunger has weakened the mind and has conquered the will, you have just devoured far more food than medically necessary to treat the surplus of insulin that has just thrown a tantrum in your body. Driven by a ruthless hunger of moments ago, you now begin to steadily climb out of the acute danger zone. But it's too late. The climb is unstoppable. And it will take you back up to that *other* place again. . . .

A few hours later, you test your blood sugar. 487. It is confirmed. You have over-treated. Again. Where you go from here depends on where you are—today. Maybe you will help your body to re-stabilize and take some extra insulin to cover over-treating. Or maybe you will just sit with it. Let the sugar stay in your blood a while and intensify. You'll feel lousy, but at least you won't gain weight from over-treating . . . . from overeating.

I wonder if they'll ever make this rollercoaster a little smoother. . . .

Speaking From Experience: Inspirations to Invite Healing

• Newton's Third Law
If you dig deep enough in your memory-bank of science lessons, you might remember learning about Newton's third law of motion: *For every action, there is an equal, opposite and collinear reaction.* Binge-purge cycles are the dietary equivalent—each behavior independently a manifestation of extreme imbalance—each one equal to the other in intensity, and opposite to the other in direction. By the way, so is yo-yo dieting.

• Extremes
Extreme actions tend to evoke extreme reactions; and extreme reactions evoke extreme reactions to the extreme reactions—and on and on and on. . . .

When I was in college I didn't own a blood glucose meter, so I had no knowledge of what my blood sugar was at any given moment. Management of my diabetes was based purely on guesswork and/or my emotional or physical response to food I had eaten, not eaten, intended to eat, or wanted to eat. If I had just driven my body through another tempestuous insulin-omission-purge for a day (or two or three), the next day I would overcompensate with insulin—20 units, 30, or sometimes even 40—all at once. The dose was based, not on calculations, but on an emotional response to my inner "bad diabetic." My velocity back toward sugar-health was directly proportionate to my perceived severity of sugar *un-health* from the previous days. At some point during the "atonement day" (the day of insulin mega-dosing) I ended up hitting the wall with a severe low blood sugar. Newton's law, anyone?

Then came insulin edema. Insulin edema is when the body bloats up like a water balloon in response to reintroducing insulin to a diabetic body following a period of hyperglycemia (high blood glucose), and I promise you, when you're addicted to feeling thin, insulin edema is pure hell! Non-clinically speaking, if yesterday had found me so dehydrated from extreme high blood sugar that my cheekbones and ribcage were protruding and my rings were sliding off my fingers, today found me plumped up so bubbly and round that my eyes disappeared behind my chubby red cheeks, and my ankles and shins felt more like model clay than human tissue—the body's response to intensive insulin therapy. It was a case of extreme dehydration followed by extreme re-hydration—extreme imbalance—on both ends. Is Newton's law screaming at you yet?

• Breaking the Cycle

Presumably, if we could avoid extremes entirely we'd avoid their toxic counterparts. But to create such expectations of perfection would risk setup for failure and self-bashing. Impulsivity promotes perpetual volatility. So what's the alternative? Break the cycle. Instead of reacting, respond. Rein in the impulse to desperately react to an extreme with another extreme and instead respond to it—deliberately, purposefully—with moderation. In short, think before acting. Consciously recognize and acknowledge the impulse to react with opposing urgency; then make the choice not to. By responding with moderation instead of reacting with impulsivity, balance will have a much easier time rediscovering its place inside you.

5

Discovering Fitness

Is That Demon Wearing a Halo?

For as long as I can remember, music has been as necessary to me as breathing. Though you can sing words to it, on its own it is wordless, a form of expression in a singular category. When I find language inadequate to express a feeling, the articulation is there in music. I sing. Then I become the music and it becomes me. We are one in the same, and right in this oneness, in this singularizing of the music and me, there is a precious opening. And in this opening, I feel God, within me and beyond me at the same time. And so, for me, music is a doorway of sorts—a doorway to something much bigger than this life.

As a child I sang, wrote, and played music. My dad and I used to spend many a summer campfire strumming guitars and making up harmonies while my younger siblings toasted marshmallows and chimed in on the refrain. I have floated from high school glee clubs and All State Choruses to community theater musicals, a capella quartettes and full circle back home to church choir. When you find something that is that vital to the thriving of your spirit, it becomes one of life's essentials—almost more essential even than *food*.

And so, I was sold on the prospect of auditioning for the Newton Country Players. It would be a blissful three months of rehearsals—in love with my art, distracted from food, and setting the stage for a boon of cardiovascular benefits (not to mention weight management benefits) from rigorous choreography sessions. It was a win-win from any angle. Life hadn't cadenced this sort of pulse since my few months at Boston Conservatory, and I was entirely drawn to it. It was like a voice inside reminding me what makes me shine from the inside out.

The first year we performed *The Wiz* and the second, *Applause*. I joined the play-reading committee and became a presence in the community theater group. Involvement in a musical production that required this level of single-minded focus was one of the only weapons to ever successfully divert me from my erratic relationship with the number line. I became so fully engaged, so distracted from the highs and lows of body-image woes, that the weight began melting off of me in buckets without any conscious effort or willpower on my part.

People were beginning to notice. Not just family and friends, people from work ("Can you write down everything you eat so I can copy it to lose weight for my wedding?"), the gym ("What exercises will give me abs like yours?"), around town, even strangers. I ran into an old musical director from college I hadn't seen in years.

"Wow!" he remarked. "You look amazing! If you'd had *that* body when we were doing *Godspell,* I would have cast you in a much bigger role."

The absolute value of thinness—confirmed in a single comment.

I have to be honest. All this attention for becoming someone I never thought I could be filled me with efficacy. And it felt great. No, it felt spectacular! I was honest-to-God thin. Really thin! For the first time since childhood. I even thought so. I knew so. (And because I recognized my own thinness, I still sometimes question the anorexia diagnosis I would receive several years later. Bulimia, okay. But anorexia? I'm not sure I'll ever completely consent to that one. Oh well, it's just a word after all. But I'm getting ahead of myself.)

One thing I loved about my new and improved body was that it didn't just happen to suddenly befall me like an unexpected gift from heaven. I was not blessed with skinny genes. I worked hard at it. *Very* hard. It was something I *accomplished*, something for which to be proud. I had become a devout fitness enthusiast, faithful to my workouts. If my schedule failed to allow me an hour to run, I'd set the alarm for 4:30 a.m. to guarantee that sacred hour of workout time. And I was fully committed to calorie shortage. I was so committed in fact that I often calculated with decimal precision the tiniest daily calorie consumption my newly shrunken body would require in order to continue its steady descent down the number line. I embraced hunger pains, reading them as a sign that fat cells were, at that very moment, actually shrinking. Not metaphorically, mind you. Physically. Scientifically.

You can be thin and healthy. What's not healthy? Physically healthy persons are not anemic, they maintain regular menstrual cycles, they have balanced nutrition, they get all their necessary vitamins, minerals, and dietary fats from food. Our culture is centered on a narrow definition of body image, and that applauds "thin" just in and of itself, and that's not always healthy.

My blood sugars responded almost poetically to this revised method of weight control, so what could be wrong with any of it? From where I stood, it looked like nothing short of a major victory.

But there is a gray space where exercise that targets health and physical fitness, and exercise that is single-mindedly fixated on calorie expenditure intersect. The boundaries of this space are vague. What was the true role of exercise in my life? Was it an access-way to good blood sugars and wellbeing, or was it in fact just another means of atonement, another tool for eradication?

One Lonely Tomato

Balance tastes sweet, but first-time success conquering the unconquerable is mouth-wateringly delicious! Engulfed in the novel flavors of such success, it is easy to get lost. And it was this newborn success, this ego-gratifying sudden attention to which I would mistakenly delegate my self-worth. It was an easy read.

We can become quite skilled at reading our bodies when we pay attention. The human body sends us clear messages all the time. We feel pain; we read, "Danger! Stop!" We experience pleasure; we read, "Good! Proceed!" We experience exhaustion; we read, "Sleep!" We experience hunger; we read "Eat!" As unmistakable as these signs are, we can also become quite good at deliberately *not* reading them.

Hunger. It begins with a whisper of sensation in the stomach. If unfed, the whisper grows to an all-out howl, audible to anyone standing in the same room. If still unfed, it transforms itself into a feeling of general emptiness and limpness, no longer isolated to the stomach but broadened to include the arms, legs, head, and even fingertips in the sensation of hollowness.

I had learned to enjoy the feeling of hunger. It translated to *"No available fuel; must go elsewhere for energy needs!"* And "elsewhere" could only be one place: body fat. Every growl, every lightheadedness, every tremor meant one thing to me—mission accomplished. If hunger meant mission accomplished, then its opposite, fullness, meant mission failed. So I learned to read my body well and I also learned to veto its instructions to me. I continuously embraced hunger as a welcome friend. Emptiness began to feel like a reward, a *high*. Just like an alcoholic wants to keep the buzz going, I wanted to keep the emptiness going. Another martini for the alcoholic. Another foodless hour for me. Hour after foodless hour can be a dangerous way for a person with diabetes to live. But I had learned so much about my body through the years and one thing I happened to stumble upon is the reality that missing a meal here and there was no more dangerous to a diabetic than it was for a non-diabetic—as long as insulin was adjusted accordingly. So if I were to miss a meal, I would reduce or miss that mealtime shot of insulin. It was pretty straightforward, almost a linear relationship. I must clarify though: This kind of insulin omission was not the same as the old kind. The objectives were practically opposite. The old way aimed for high blood sugars in order to promote *ketoacidosis* for fat loss, attacking that blood sugar goal from both ends: excessive food, zero insulin. This new way was aimed at keeping insulin levels low enough to ensure food-intake could also remain low.

There comes a point however, when a coveted feeling of emptiness crosses the line of sweet success to all-consuming debilitation. From a whisper to a howl to a generalized emptiness—to an insufferable headache. That's when you know your body is hauling you over the coals, reprimanding you for pushing it over the borderline. You wonder how long you can withstand the pounding agony before something crashes and brings you to the threshold where you've stood many times—the one where you cave in to the recklessness and urgency of a binge. The binge—a sudden hero that rescues you from the hellish fires of starvation. In the moment you begin, you know where it's going to lead you. But this kind of binge is much different than a mindless surrender to the temptation of a forbidden decadence. It is a binge of physical desperation for fuel. So it begins with something as innocent as—a single tomato.

And that's exactly how it started one Saturday afternoon in late August. One lonely tomato fresh from Dad's garden. Whole. Red. Juicy. Succulent. Sweet. . . . removed from a brown paper bag he had given us a few days earlier when we had visited him for his birthday. His crop had yielded too many for one solo divorcee to eat all by himself. He didn't know what to do with all of them so we departed with a goodie-bag filled to the brim. How many were there? I didn't count them, but I know for a fact there were more than nine. . . . because though I didn't count them in the bag, I absolutely counted each and every one that passed through my lips.

When you have crossed the great divide between the triumphant buzz of emptiness and the excruciating throb of torment banging from inside your temples, when you are standing in the middle of hunger's loudest hour, nine ripe tomatoes seasoned lightly with salt and pepper is delicious paradise without a single thread of guilt—until you begin adding up the calories, one juicy tomato at a time. Weighing in at 22 calories each I had just consumed nearly 200 calories of nutrient dense vegetation. That might have been perfectly acceptable *if* it had been intended as a meal. But it was three o'clock in the afternoon—too late for lunch, too early for dinner. We would need to "take care" of this somehow.

Well fine then, I resolved swiftly, unemotionally, and without much inner deliberation. No need to wonder what dinner would be today. I had just eaten it.

This was pretty much how I continued to keep things "under control" for a while. A long while I suppose. If I ate something at a time or in an amount that did not conform to whatever diet rules I happened to be committed to at the time, then I would repay the extra calories in some way at the next meal or during the next workout. I kept meticulous mental records of my calorie budget and I was very good about reimbursement whenever I was overdrawn. I was completely unstoppable. I had all the tools I needed. I even stuffed one of those exercise bands into my suitcase once on a vacation to ensure access to my workout. I could go as far as I wanted to go. . . .

And I wanted to go far. Very far. I wanted to take it all the way to the limit, or at least to discover where that limit really existed. And the scale dropped from 112 to 108 to 105 . . . . to 105 . . . . to 105 . . . .

Like a broken record! I was stuck at one hundred-five pounds for what felt like eternity. I calculated calories, measured and weighed all my food, ran harder and faster—and then sprained an ankle. But it didn't stop me.

Crutches are awfully tiresome. They demand extraordinary upper body strength. So even though life's circumstances kept me off the road, I could still use up extra calories by requiring my upper body to take up some of the slack for a while. That's when I invented a new workout—laps around the house—on crutches. Then came the chafing under the armpits, and I had to stop.

But it was only a few weeks of exercise-less torture before I was back in the game, counting, measuring, running, lifting, weighing. . . .

102! Finally unstuck, I was released from the quicksand of 105! Victory at last! So where do you go from a victory? To the next victory, of course.

As I scrutinized and dissected my abs in the mirror, my eyes immediately fixated on that one pocket of fleshiness around my lower section. How many more pounds would I need to lose to get rid of *that?* I eyeballed that one section and mentally likened it to the size of a three-pound raw chicken breast. The early years of weighing every morsel of food I ate to be sure it was a perfect fit for my diabetic meal plan had trained me well. Now a master eyeballer, I could accurately transpose almost any food into the equivalent value of another. Half a grapefruit could become 12 grapes or an unsweetened popsicle; three cups of popcorn could become one slice of whole wheat bread; one egg could become one-quarter cup of cottage cheese—and a three pound chicken breast could become a tiny bulge protruding just beneath my navel. I had grown so accustomed to exchanging one food for another that my conversions had become nearly flawless. This unusual talent I owe to the conditioning of my early diabetic years.

Yes, three pounds would take care of it. Three more pounds and maybe I could have the abs of. . . .

Who? Whose abs did I want anyway? And if I could answer that question, then I'd have to ask the next one: Why? And then. . . .

Deeper.

Go deeper, girl! WHY?

But I couldn't answer.

A New Key to an Old Place

I'd long since stopped using insulin manipulation as my primary tool for weight management. This is not to say that I stopped seeking permanent membership in The Skinny Club, simply that I adjusted the means to that end. I don't recall making a *decision* to stop exactly; I just stopped. Conversely, *decision* itself had everything to do with a lifestyle of fitness that had now taken on a rhythm of its own. I had invited it to come into my world and stay for good. Intense exercise—tons of it—had craftily tiptoed in to take over as the new purge. So though I was still as fixated on shrinking every cubic inch of personal anatomy below my eyebrows as I'd always been, the bathroom scale had become one of my new BFFs, dependable about spoon-feeding me daily nuggets of affirmation. It was a time when I'd been teaching countless fitness classes a week and running at least two hours every weekend, so the insurmountable battle of the bulge had started to feel much more accommodating and cooperative. I concluded that my calling to this fitness lifestyle turned out to be the key that unlocked the door to the possibility of developing a body I'd wished for in a darker time. Was I cured of my evil ways—the insulin-omission-purge—for good, or just in remission?

I was enrolled in a fitness convention and master's class for credit toward my recertification. The auditorium-sized studio for the affair was crowded with fellow group exercise instructors and fitness professionals eagerly attempting to master the instructor's choreography. These events reliably offered a complete banquet of both men and women with amazingly sculpted shapes and lean physiques, which had a way of causing my all-consuming sense of body consciousness to swell.

As I struggled to perfect my footing in the choreography, I indiscriminately scanned the mirror in the front of the studio. My eyes aimlessly wandered across mobs of magnificently fit bodies when I suddenly honed in on a set of six-pack abs that appeared notably chiseled. I respected them from my distant vantage point and I remember briefly wondering if my still relatively young commitment to this world of fitness might ever afford me the opportunity to achieve such a degree of triumph. These musings took me all but a few nanoseconds before I noticed that the torso I happened to be inspecting—or dissecting—was my very own.

Perhaps the imperfections I'd noticed in this morning's mirror—a mere two feet in front of me—were now camouflaged by the additional space between the studio mirror and me. Or maybe not. Maybe I had arrived. Or at the very least maybe I'd finally begun to approach the person I'd always wanted to be—on the outside.

Speaking From Experience: Inspirations to Invite Healing

• **Have You Heard the Secret?**
I doubt there's anyone alive on the planet today who hasn't heard the "secret" but I'll say it out loud once more, just in case: *EXERCISE IS IMPERATIVE TO OUR HEALTH!* We know this already, but

somewhere along the line of coming to believe it, I fear the rationale at the core of its truth has become gravely overlooked.

In my 25+ years of work in fitness, the advice solicited from me most often is the answer to one question: "What's the best (or easiest, or quickest) way to lose X pounds?" But the *real* value of exercise proudly stands miles and miles outside the perimeter of its calorie-burning benefits. It is the one and only antidote to the pestilences of 21st century modernized living.

• Fourscore and Seven Centuries Ago

For our ancestors, the physical demands of heavy weightlifting and intense cardio workouts were built into everyday life. Grueling physical work was essential for every inning of the survival game from food and shelter to transportation and recreation. They had no access to local take-out huts for those "to-go" dinners. For them eating meant tilling the soil, farming the land, chopping wood, stalking prey and killing beasts—in short, the kind of nonstop physical demands comparable to those of an Ironman triathlon. But today's modern world has "rescued" us from all this backbreaking work.

No doubt the modernization of our planet is a formidable testament to the success of our species, but it is also simultaneously our curse. While humanity's worldly progress has afforded us a wealth of pragmatic luxuries, consider the true cost of these conveniences, namely the plagues of inactivity—obesity, heart disease, cancer, hypertension, osteoporosis, memory loss, arthritis, depression—and diabetes just to name a few. Life no longer necessitates physical labor for basic survival. Consequently, we are laden with disease.

• Back to the Basic Nature of Things

Just because arduous physical work is no longer necessary for *immediate* survival doesn't mean it's not essential for long-term survival and wellbeing. But enough about the survival benefits. There is a value to exercise that far supersedes winning at the survival game.

Consider children. Before they ever discover T.V. and videogames they innately move nonstop around their spaces (hence the invention of those plastic child-gates). Could it possibly be that nature *wanted* us to be physical?

Do you recall those long bike rides of childhood, those late summer afternoon dips in the lake, jumping rope for hours or finally making it to the tippitty-top of the jungle gym? Do you remember the sizzle of childhood energy that circulated in your blood during those neighborhood kickball games and relay races on the front lawn? Or maybe you find it more meaningful to reminisce about racing ahead of the pack during one of those family hiking trips. Now, dig deep. Do you remember the joy and vigor that remained with you for hours afterward?

• For the Joy of it
There is great evidence that exercise not only bolsters fitness gains and calorie expenditure, but our joy barometers as well. What could be the link between physical exertion and joy? Might it be that in those moments, we catch whispers of a much deeper domain of wellbeing where body and spirit intersect and unify?

We are designed for movement, and if our culture by and large continues to defy Nature's intent, I fear that Darwin's theory of Natural Selection may one day have its way with the human species.

Saying yes to exercise is a no-brainer, but not because of what it does for our figures. May I suggest that we stop fixating on those digital calorie-counters on the cardio machines at the gym and instead aim to rediscover our innateness—movement for the pure *joy* of it.

6

Battling Infertility

A Different War

I was always looking for some form of the "clean slate." Anything is possible when you're standing at the beginning of a new road.

One of my favorite pastimes when I was a little girl was playing dress-up. I could be anyone I wanted to be. There were no borders on my imagination. I loved playing dolls too. Loved being the mom. I used to set up an entire living space in my playroom for my pretend family, complete with Susie-homemaker oven, miniature table and chairs, and doll-sized beds for my "children" constructed from shoeboxes, scraps of fabric, and tissue-stuffed pillows. My pretend family life had become so real to me then that I could never bear to part with the do-it-yourself photo albums I had crafted one rainy afternoon, from stapled together pieces of paper sketched with drawings of my favorite dolls. I was so proud of those photo albums that I think they might actually still be somewhere tucked away in the attic along with the dolls themselves.

During the first several years of our marriage, Russ and I spent many a Sunday afternoon sitting around my mother-in-law's kitchen table sipping coffee and nibbling on Italian treats. (Well . . . . *they* nibbled on the treats. *I* just sipped coffee . . . . *most* of the time.) Together we enjoyed musing about a wide range of subjects, but one of our most regularly visited topics was a very specific lusted fantasy—of parenthood for Russ and me, and grand-motherhood for her. She repeatedly retrieved a particular aged baby photo of Russ, as if by fixing her eyes upon it again and again had the power to magically transport her to a place where she might relive the treasured moments of those years. The photo was a true prizewinner in fact, a beautiful black-and-white that was once displayed in the window of Grover Cronin's department store. My mother-in-law's admiration was entirely justified. Her son, my husband, really was a beautiful child. Together we created delightful fantasies of our future family, bonding over the "someday" prospect of my bringing one of my own little *Russells* into this world.

I very much enjoyed our pleasant Sunday afternoons with my new extended family. Life was feeling pretty okay these days. Predictable. Doable. Stable. Dreamy. Fun. Routine—but not boring. Russ and I decided it was time to begin figuring out when we would start working on a family. We both had jobs. We owned a home. Nothing extravagant, but charming with a fenced-in backyard. There's never a perfect time, but anytime can be the right time.

I always loved children. I wanted them for my own. Life seemed to be grooming me for motherhood practically since the day I was born: the oldest of six, a perpetual babysitter, even an early childhood major in college. But pregnancy? Was I okay with that part of it? I had finally gotten to a point where my weight was just beginning to approach "acceptable"—not quite there yet, but almost. Pregnancy meant weight *gain*. How could I tolerate something so extremely counterproductive to all that I aimed to become? I'd spent my entire life trying so hard to go the opposite direction. If I succeeded in becoming pregnant, expansion would be unstoppable. I would be mandated to drive the wrong way down a one-way street—at full-speed!

I marinated in the vision of a pregnant me. There was a wide range of pregnant bodies to envision. Some of them were actually kind of cute, I had to admit to myself. But there was no guarantee I'd turn out to wear pregnancy like one of them. There was the body whose arms and face look just as pregnant as the belly. My imagination offered me a vision of a woman with overgrown hair, no makeup, oily skin, and wrinkled clothes. Sweaty, bloated, unkempt and clearly uncomfortable. Then I considered the opposite—a well-dressed woman with an edgy haircut, tall, thin, and fashionable, glamorously made-up with a cute little beach-ball-shaped belly and two pencil thin legs connecting the adorable beach-ball-belly to the floor. Maybe if I was exceptionally careful with my calories, I could be the beach-ball lady. I hoped, but I was so afraid. Nature didn't seem to be on my side for this one.

And what about my diabetes? Here I was worrying about what pregnancy would *look* like, when I ought to be considering the real issues— blindness, kidney disease, stroke, amputations . . . . I was terrified. But at the same time, I was too excited about the potential for actualizing my childhood dreams to *not* try. So I created a neat little denial pile for all of my fears. And I refused to look at that pile until life had its way with me—whatever that meant.

I began to "notice" my first signs of pregnancy after our very first month of trying. I was sure the days of practice-parenthood with my childhood baby dolls would at long last come to pay out its dividends within the year . . . . but apparently I was very good at imagining my own feeling of nausea.

After a year of not conceiving, we decided to see a specialist. Russ was fine. His "little fish" were abounding with energy, strong enough to swim against a tidal wave. It was my fault. Of course it was. *My* body's fault we couldn't get pregnant. Maybe this was my punishment for all those years of using and abusing my body as a tool to fill my selfish need for the shallowest degree of personal value a person could seek.

Infertility workups were slow and grueling. Some things had to be ruled out before others could be ruled in. It was a needle in a haystack, or more like a single needle in ten thousand haystacks. Then there was the waiting game. I became a human research project for countless specialists who worked tirelessly trying to figure out the inner workings of my broken body. And then, just when they would begin to get somewhere, without any provocation, my body would simply decide to take a break from ovulating, and all progress would stagnate until the break was over. Sometimes that meant waiting two or three months. But science had come so very far and answers began to unfold in tiny increments for my dedicated team of specialists.

It was a cumbersome undertaking, demanding weekly and sometimes even daily appointments at Boston IVF. All of my emotional energy was attached to it. My focus at my full-time office job waned, as did my attendance. I was overlooked for promotions and continually reprimanded for my poor attendance record. Admittedly I felt defensive. And then I felt worthless.

And one Friday night after an upsetting annual review, for the first time in years, I binged on chocolate chip cookie dough. And then I purged—the old way—the high-sugar-food-hangover way. My old "friend," self-hate didn't take long to respond to my invitation and this time she returned with a presence louder than an Aerosmith rock concert. How could I have done something like this in the throes of trying to conceive? But I did. I wanted to give up—on all of it. Maybe I just wasn't supposed to have children. Maybe I wasn't supposed to be happy. Ever.

It would take four years of appointments with infertility specialists, four years of early morning blood tests, four years of hormone shots and surgeries and procedures, four years of disappointment, before I would experience my first real pregnancy. Russ and I sat anxiously on the phone, he in the den, I in the kitchen, waiting to hear that magical number—the number that represented the quantity of beta sub cells in my blood. . . .

We were pregnant. The beta sub number was even higher than the doctors had hoped. We told everyone. Why wait? They had traveled this miserable infertility journey with us for the past four years, supporting us, consoling us, distracting us from our despair. They all deserved to share in our victory.

Six weeks later, we got to hear the heartbeat . . . . heartbeat . . . . heart*beat?* I mean . . . . *heartbeats!* There were *two!* We were going to have twins! We were beside ourselves with gratitude and excitement. We were convinced we were on the brink of an all-inclusive parent package deal—a life of not just toy fire engines and little league games, but pink lace, ballet recitals and Barbie dolls too. We had names all picked out, Andrew and Amanda. One boy, one girl—the perfect family!

Two weeks later, another ultrasound . . . . only *one* heartbeat. Our hearts sank, but we clung desperately to the hope for the remaining life still hanging on inside me. The doctors checked my numbers every day. They were supposed to be doubling now. We followed up religiously. But the numbers weren't doubling. They weren't even increasing. They called me in for another ultrasound. And there it was. The bleakest of truths. No heartbeat.

The D and C was scheduled for the following morning. . . .

Miscarriage is the most common complication of early pregnancy.

As anyone who has ever suffered a miscarriage knows, the experience of this loss was as real as the death of a loved one. It was absolutely devastating. Maybe we had never gotten to look upon those infants' faces, or feel their miniature fingers wrapped around ours, or see their tiny lips pursed around the nipple of a baby bottle, but those babies had existed. They had been as real to me, to us, as the ground we walk on, as real as love, as real as hope. And as anyone who has experienced the loss of an unborn baby also knows, when that life inside you—that non-actualized possibility of family, that hope—ceases to exist, a piece of you dies too.

Perhaps the true function of the roadblocks in our lives is not to keep us from reaching the other side, but to help us to define for ourselves how important it is to get there. I would have four more miscarriages, three more IVF's, countless progesterone shots, two occasions of severely hyper-stimulated ovaries requiring a week's bed-rest each time, and oceans upon oceans of tears during the next two years before finally finding real hope for the possibility of motherhood.

Green Faces and Butterflies

I was a silent whiner during pregnancy. I didn't need to say a word. My facial posture and body language said it all. Morning sickness set in almost immediately. It was undeniably miles from pleasant, but I felt so extraor-dinarily grateful to experience it for real this time that I *invited* it to stay regardless. How was I to expect it would overstay its welcome by such a huge margin? Russ was diligent about his 'nightly target practice' whereby my buttocks served as a fleshy bull's-eye and progesterone-filled intramus-cular syringes (the huge ones!) were transformed into shooting darts. Ultra-sounds and blood tests became a bi-weekly routine and by week five, both confirmed optimum progress—and another *twin* pregnancy.

Pregnancy clinic at Joslin Diabetes Center was every Tuesday morn-ing. I met with a new team of specialists each week, among them obste-tricians, endocrinologists, nephrologists, ophthalmologists, nutritionists, teaching nurses, even the occasional psychologist (just in case). My blood sugars were routinely evaluated; my kidneys and eyes were watched care-fully for vascular leakage and protein spillage; my bodyweight was me-ticulously monitored and recorded, my eating habits were discussed, my abdomen measured . . . . It was a medical circus!

It is now possible for women with Type 1 Diabetes to expect a successful pregnancy resulting in a healthy baby, with minor or no complications for the mother. But a successful pregnancy with diabetes does require extra planning and effort. This is largely due to tight blood sugar control, which requires frequent daily blood sugar monitoring and insulin adjustment.

I continued working my fulltime hours at the insurance company and continued teaching fitness classes at the gym nights. I secretly hoped that Dr. Greene, my obstetrician would strongly encourage me to discontinue one or both, however. I was pushing fatigue considerably further than I was used to, and now without the incentive of weight loss. But he offered no such suggestion. It was "good for my blood sugar and good for my general well-being." I'd promised myself I wouldn't slow down until the order came in the form of medical advice so I persevered through fitness classes and office work, fully equipped with a personal supply of nausea-combative saltines at all times.

"Your face is looking a little . . . . *green*," my supervisor noticed one morning. Moments later my race to the restroom caused nothing short of a windstorm.

The nausea was growing exponentially. Perhaps it was because I had 'double the trouble' growing inside, twice the embryos I might have otherwise produced had science not needed to be involved. Perhaps it was the mega-doses of nightly progesterone Russ was shooting into my buttocks, both to demolish the embryo toxins my body was producing and to prevent a sixth miscarriage. Perhaps the years of self-induced vomiting were taking their toll on my digestion. I couldn't know the reason, but the reality was unmistakable. I was pregnant and I had gotten here intentionally. And this morning sickness was not too eager to vacate the premises. It apparently felt perfectly entitled to show up unannounced—at *any* time of day.

Once at a stoplight, I urgently shoved open the car door to prevent having a 'disaster' right inside my car; another time I had to leave a customer on hold while I flew into the restroom in a panic. Nearly every day at the end of the rush hour commute home, I frenziedly bee-lined to the half-bath in the basement of our home before even removing my coat. I recalled the days of binge-purge self-induced vomiting and I thought, I must have been absurdly mad to have ever caused this process *on purpose*. Now in gross discomfort, I vowed I would never do *that* again.

It was Tuesday morning again. (It was *always* Tuesday morning.) I'd just begun week 13 of my pregnancy. Two strong heartbeats, one very strong urge to vomit, and one swollen body . . . . Time for the weekly weigh-in.

"And now ladies and gentlemen," announced the nurse as if entertaining a nonexistent audience, "the grand total for trimester one—*13 pounds!*"

Oh no! I thought. That's an average of a pound a week. Nobody gains weight at this rate until the third trimester! Some women actually *lose* weight in their first trimester. I'd hoped to be one of those women. You would have thought that all that nausea would have been useful for *something*. At this rate, I was going to be bigger than the continent before I was finished!

My body did not yet *look* pregnant. But it did look fat. I was definitely not the "beach ball lady." I hated my body again. And worse—all this nausea was reminding me of my days of skipping insulin and *ketoacidosis* madness. Get over yourself! I thought. It's nine months. Man up, girl! You've gone through much worse, playing for a far lesser prize. But nine months felt like a lifetime.

. . . . until the day I felt something like a butterfly fluttering inside of me. Or was it an alien? Maybe just gas. Nope. Definitely not gas. This was a new feeling. I called my mother-in-law right away to describe my sensation in detail and elicit her assessment. Her diagnosis was immediate. No question about it. The babies were moving. This butterfly or alien became my new reality. And in the moments observing waves ripple across my abdomen, moments pressing against those waves to feel them pressing back, Russ and I began our relationship with our unseen children. It was then that we chose their names, Travis and Taylor.

I was 26 weeks into my pregnancy. I asked Dr. Greene how long I'd be able to continue teaching my step classes? It was a question I managed to sneak in every time I met with him. (Please . . . . tell me to stop now! Remember I'm a high-risk pregnancy. I have twins in here! I'm diabetic. I'm not even *supposed* to be pregnant. Nature didn't get me this way. *We* did. You and me and medical technology! I'm only in this state because of the miracle science of the era into which I happened to be born . . . . the infertility itself makes me high-risk even without any of my other risk factors. What are you waiting for? I'm *exhausted!!)*

"How do you feel?" It was the first time my comfort was even a factor in the medical answer to my secret plea for permission to rest.

"Exhausted," I answered honestly.

"Your blood-pressure is a little elevated and you're beginning to spill small amounts of protein in your urine," he finally conceded. "Why don't you begin to take it easy."

The long-awaited "permission" to surrender to my fatigue had finally arrived. I gave my notice to the gym and had finally earned the luxury of indulging myself in the peaceful laziness of sitting around eating ice cream and watching sitcoms—guilt free! It was doctor's orders after all! I was still throwing up every day, but food had finally decided to give me a few occasional moments of pleasure again too. I'd made temporary peace with ice cream and my inner couch potato now. I was on so much insulin that neither had much effect on my blood sugars and I had finally resigned myself to the inevitability of my ballooning body. Obsession was a greedy energy-eater and I was growing more fatigued by the minute. Obsession would have to wait.

A "Sophie's" Choice

It was July 20, 1993. And it was Tuesday—again. I'd been confined to bed rest for the past month, allowed to be vertical only for the few moments needed to walk from my bed to the bathroom or eat a meal. Tuesdays and Fridays however I was exempt from these restrictions. In addition to the Tuesday Pregnancy Clinic at Joslin, Fridays had become my regular day for non-stress tests. I knew the drill well. Blood test first; then leave my specimen of urine; then weigh-in; then the blood pressure; then the Joslin endocrinologist; then Dr. Greene, the obstetrician.

"You feeling tired?" He never started this way. Yes, I was most definitely feeling tired. But I was always tired these days. Today was no different. "I think you're going to be joining us today."

Okay, there goes my heart. Loud . . . . louder . . . . faster . . . . I wonder if Dr. Greene can *hear* it.

My blood pressure and kidneys were doing worse this week. My protein was elevated. I had pre-eclampsia and needed round-the-clock care and monitoring.

And for the next five days, I became a human extension chord—from one piece of medical equipment to the next—non-stress tests, ultrasounds, monitors, daily amniocenteses . . . . *more* blood tests! 'Come on! I *must* be running out of blood by now!'

On Monday morning, July 26, after Sunday's amniocentesis and ultrasound were evaluated, Dr. Greene came into my room with the pregnancy version of *Sophie's Choice*. The amnio had shown that Travis' lungs were not yet mature and therefore it would be better for *him* to remain in-utero a little longer. The ultrasound had shown that Taylor's movement was slowing perilously and if we did not deliver promptly, *she* may be stillborn.

The overwhelming powerlessness of that single moment defies words. Were we truly expected to be capable of making such an enormous decision based on our limited medical understanding of the possible outcomes? Choice is a powerful right, a human right. But this was not a choice we were capable of owning. We were ill equipped to make it.

God never gives us more than we can handle, someone once said. Maybe what happened next helped me to believe in the truth of that statement.

That afternoon, Dr. Greene entered my hospital room with the results of the morning's amnio. Travis' lungs had matured enough to withstand delivery. And, on Monday night, July 26, 1993, my entire world changed—forever.

Speaking From Experience: Inspirations to Invite Healing

• Do You Believe in Miracles?

I'm sure you'll find it easy to comprehend why motherhood was for me the greatest of all miracles—first to be told by nature and science that all I had ever hoped or expected to become was not to be, not ever; then to be inhabited for 36 weeks by what felt like alien creatures moving inside me; and then, at the end of it all, feeling my soul becoming entirely absorbed into the most overwhelming, all-consuming kind of love I had ever known. Miracle. It was the only word for it.

What exactly does that word "miracle" mean? Some say it's an act of God; some that it's an event that defies the laws of nature; some say it's simply something entirely unexpected and amazing, possibly even magical. Others will say that miracles do not exist anywhere other than in fantasy.

Whether or not you believe in miracles will largely depend on how you define them and how that definition fits into your own experience. I've come to define a miracle as when something extraordinary is manifested in the ordinary. It shows up in countless varieties of shapes, sizes, forms, and venues. It is, at its root essence, a gift—from God, from science, from nature, from life.

• Miracle of the Human Body

Can we not find the miracle in the idea of trillions of cells and systems working together in perfect synchronicity to perform such marvels as breathing, moving, growing, thinking, seeing, reproducing, emoting, nourishing, regenerating, healing, living? Consider the anatomy: lungs that inflate and deflate automatically, minute-by-minute to extract life-sustaining oxygen from an atmosphere where oxygen comprises only 21% of the total composite; a small sac of striated muscle tissue called the heart no bigger than a mere tennis-ball contracting and releasing rhythmically almost three billion times during its life in order to circulate liters of nourishing blood through a vast network of arteries and veins to exactly where and exactly when that nourishment is needed; an immune system that sends out volumes of white cells to protect and defend the wellbeing and functionality of our anatomy by recognizing and neutralizing damaging pathogens and free radicals.

Our bodies serve and protect us every day—in ways we see and in ways we don't see. What if we could just stop all the judging and dissecting once and for all, and instead purposefully choose to search the far corners of our hearts for one tiny sliver of compassion, gratitude and utter amazement toward these underappreciated conglomerates of organs, cells, impulses, and systems that work day after day, arduously, seamlessly, sometimes against all odds, to make living possible? What if we could do that, just decide, right now, to respect and honor the gift that has been bequeathed to us, to marvel in it and nourish it, to celebrate it, to love it? Do you think that might be possible?

7

Motherhood

"Newby"

The first weeks of motherhood were as demanding as they were cherished. Still recovering from the physical stress of a c-section, I made daily trips with Russ to the neonatal intensive care unit where both infants still needed more "baking" time in incubators. I began to acclimate myself to the logistics of breastfeeding two preemies whose mouths were still too premature (so the nurses said) to be fully successful with sucking and latching. And then came . . . . The Pump! The $800 monster that looked like it ought to be attached to a cow somewhere on a dairy farm in the Midwest instead of a human rookie mom like me.

My choice to breastfeed had a couple of layers to it. First, my mom had breastfed all of my siblings and me for extended periods of our infanthood and I was programmed to believe in its merits—the mother-child bonding value, the superior caliber of nourishment, the benefits of an improved immune system for infants who consumed it. For all of those reasons, I'd already decided that Mom was right. But there was a secret incentive for me as well, though I'm honestly ashamed to admit to it. I had read that breastfeeding burns an additional six hundred calories a day. What a bonus! I could give my two newborns the start they deserved while getting back in shape at the same time. It was a win-win.

Here is where I began to teach cardio kick boxing classes at the ungodly hour of 5:30 A.M. two mornings a week. On the other days, I was free to choose a more rational hour for a workout but at least this new commitment would behoove me to get in shape again without detracting from quality bonding time with my new twins. During the ten weeks following Travis and Taylor's birth, I toggled between persistent attempts at breastfeeding and pumping, cardio workouts before sunrise, kissing and stroking the baby-soft skin on the faces of my new arrivals, diaper changing, running, and. . . .

Here in the middle of all of it, were these two untouched, beautifully innocent blossoms of nature and medicine. Tiny. Magnificent. It was all so amazing to behold. They had arrived without instructions, without blueprints or diagrams. And yet nature was telling them exactly what they needed and when they needed it—when to cry, when to suck, when to sleep, when to poop . . . . and when to do it all over again. It was the sweetest mix of stress and euphoria.

Motherhood. It is life changing. It is hope and possibility. It is challenge and renewal. It is precious. And it is entirely pivotal. About-face pivotal! One hundred eighty degrees pivotal! U-turn pivotal! When life gives you a gift this enormous, a purpose this essential, it has a uniquely singular way of asking you to look deeper inside, to see what is real, to define that for which you stand. Motherhood is a question to which the answer does not arrive in a single moment, but in many installments. It is a process, a journey.

Innovation's Giggles

Travis and Taylor were calling all the shots now. They had dwindled down to two naps a day and, if I do say so myself, they were a bit inconsiderate about communicating their 'nap-plans' to me—and to each other! A nap could be anywhere from thirty minutes for one and three hours for the other (or vice-versa), to two hours of unexpected silence—for the entire house. But it took a long time for me to be bothered by the inconsistency. I was purely infatuated with my life in this new role.

Maternity leave was a dual blessing. First and foremost was the blessing of motherhood itself. I adored all the quiet hours of sitting and watching my babies absorbing their new world. There was nothing sweeter than seeing them learn to smile, or learn that hitting the squeeze-toy could evoke a sound; nothing sweeter than seeing two babies prone on a blanket one minute and in the next instant witnessing the astonishment of a first rollover; nothing sweeter than finding them find each other—making eye contact first and then body contact second. (I remember once giggling when I found a finger of one in the mouth of the other.) And there was absolutely nothing sweeter than looking into the eyes of innocence and feeling the embrace of recognition, gratitude, and unchangeable love.

In addition to all the wonderfulness of motherhood, maternity leave also bestowed upon me a secondary blessing: a much-needed respite from the full-time office world I had come to loathe. I so dreaded the prospect of needing to return to that world once my leave was over and I prayed that I might discover some unknown part-time position waiting for someone with just my credentials to fill it—a fitness job perhaps that paid an actual salary; some unknown hero of a health and fitness facility to liberate me from the golden handcuffs of a stressful (and personally empty and unfulfilling) full-time insurance career. It was my customized version of nearly every working mom's secret fantasy. There was only one thing that truly mattered now. Everything I needed from life was now right here in front of me. Well, at least I still had several months ahead of me to live in this glorious fantasy world before maternity leave would bring this dream to an end.

In November, however, when the view beyond the family room window foreshadowed a season of lost aliveness and fading sunlight, cabin fever hit without notice. My fitness routine, which had become centered on running in the crisp autumn air with Travis and Taylor snuggled into the jogger's stroller, had now become suddenly contained and confined. Inactivity was beginning to gnaw at my insides as I envisioned fat cells accumulating around my entire torso. We were a one-car family at this point and it was much too cold to bring tiny ones outdoors at this time of year. The naptime-jogtime ritual had become my reprieve from both isolation and inactivity since their birth. Now with winter fast approaching, if I was not scheduled to teach at the gym on a particular day, my options for a workout were somewhat limited. I loved motherhood with every molecule of my being, but I had reinvented myself as a fitness devotee well before pregnancy, and this new purpose was not going to become an excuse to abandon the lifestyle that had rescued me from a world of sugar highs and food hangovers.

Desperate for exercise, I released my creativity and began exploring new frontiers of physical output. It was this very desperation that would give birth to my invention for maximizing calorie expenditure. It was simple. It was affordable. It could be done during naptime right on the premises. It was a fitness panacea for the winter blues. Drum roll please. . . . The Deck-Climb. With a five-pound dumbbell in each hand and baby monitor on the porch turned up full volume, I climbed the deck stairway, two steps at a time in ten-minute intervals. Then, to break it up a bit for both interest and muscle variation, I jumped rope for five minutes. Each pair of alternating intervals lasted a total of fifteen minutes and I did this for an hour. Naptime had taken on a whole new meaning. I'm sure the neighbors had a few laughs over the ludicrousness of my inventive and unrelenting determination, but it really worked for me. I couldn't have kept weight on if I *wanted* to! I was back at the top of my game again.

There is only one thing dependable about the duration of infants' naptimes—the undependability of them. I was thirty-five minutes into my afternoon workout one day when the baby monitor resonated with the familiar music of Travis' cry. I rushed quietly into the nursery and immediately scooped him from his crib to prevent him from waking his sister, the light-sleeper. I was still heavily layered in both inner and outerwear and the sweat-drenched t-shirt was beginning to adhere to my skin. My heart and lungs could not forget that they remained in the throes of an endorphin-producing cardio zone and the rhythmic breathing they cadenced set an ideal tempo for Travis' prompt removal from the nursery. Fully knowledgeable of the risks of abruptly halting a workout of this intensity, I whisked my son into the family room where I continued to move briskly. I was still holding Travis close as I slowed to basic squats and his crying slowed to random baby coos. The background sound of the radio provided a pulsing beat with which to work.

Then I heard it for the very first time—the sound that would make me smile all the way down inside my big toe. It was a sound that escaped his miniature mouth unintentionally, unassumingly. And this young beautiful sound was unmistakable. It was a tiny adorable giggle. Innovation's giggle coming straight from the bottom of my tiny son's belly. I squatted again. The sound repeated. Then I squatted with emphasis and exaggeration. At first, the tender giggle repeated; then a crescendo of laughter; and within seconds, I was laughing too. I don't know how long the very first moment of Travis' laughter lasted, but I'll never forget that it began in his sweat-drenched, cardio engorged mother's arms.

Monster Movie

I was beginning to get it—this idea of balance. I wasn't there yet. But I was learning. Maybe motherhood is the impetus that made me *need* to learn. It was Survival of the Fittest (pun . . . . *intended*). A sort of Balance Darwinism, I guess. Swim or drown. Defeat or be defeated. Learn how to survive or die (or let *it* kill you). What is *it?* Life—the incalculable demands; the immeasurable joys; the outrageous neuroses; the unyielding regrets; the endless obstacle course; the limitless growth; the work; the play; the laughter; the tears; the shame; the pride. Just life. All of it. It can swallow you up whole and spit you out in tiny little pieces—or not. It's up to us. It was up to me.

If there's one thing I've learned about balance, it's this: Don't get too comfortable when you get there because something's bound to come in and tip the scales. Usually it's more than one thing. I mean one thing is easy to offset. Two things might even be manageable. But several essential factors simultaneously converging at a single point, when that point marks your critical and fragile center of gravity . . . . it's guaranteed to stir your equilibrium.

Motherhood challenges even the most stable among us. Why? Because once we enter into it, it's inherently the most essential function we own. And we know this intuitively. It's entirely up to us to fill these tiny absorbent sponges with a well-designed set of principles by which to guide them to fit into a world whose rules were cemented in place long before their existence had even come to be imagined. Everything that used to be important becomes background noise in comparison. And if you happen to find yourself standing in a place of uncertainty, questioning the merit of some of the very principles you are painstakingly aiming to impart, the uncertainty itself becomes an added stressor.

I was beginning to find my work environment at the insurance company unbearable. For me, my job was one enormous, utterly meaningless pit of stress. But then there was the important piece of my world: my joy; my reason; my fuel. Travis and Taylor were now two. Exploring, playing, learning, growing, making messes and testing limits . . . . needing. As anyone who has ever parented a two-year-old knows, it is a trying phase of parenting by any standards. It wears on your patience, your stamina, your composure—and it is exhausting. But this was my purpose now. And it was worth every morsel of energy and investment that it demanded of me.

I'm not so egocentric as to believe that I could possibly be the only mother alive to experience the challenge of the working mom's juggling act. Nor do I assume for a moment that my burdens were anything out of the ordinary. I personally know many moms that have juggled a lot more than I, and quite successfully, at least to the naked eye. But we all have our thresholds. We stretch our boundaries as far as possible. And if it's not far enough, or we *think* it's not far enough to satisfy the needs of the moment and deem us valuable human beings. . . .

I can't honestly remember the trigger for what I'm about to describe. I don't even think there was one. It was more of a cumulative effect of struggling to balance all of it—the day-to-day self-imposed standards of motherhood, the personal commitment to climb to the top of the fitness ladder, the unpredictability of my blood sugars, the accelerated demands of a progressing workplace—the various pieces of life that seemed important—important either because I valued them authentically, or because I felt as though I *should* value them. When everything is *that* important—even if it isn't really—something's going to pay a price.

I was no longer in control of my own life. But if I wasn't, who or what was? My kids? My job? My fickle blood sugars? My commitment to work out no matter what? They all took their turn. And then there was food. The abundance of it. The lure of it. The self-imposed deprivation of it. Oh sure, I was proud of how strong my willpower had grown in recent years but that didn't mean the temptation itself had ever quieted down. It was always there, whether center stage or fading into the background. It never went away. I just became very good at ignoring it. But when limits extend and demands push, weakness is sure to resurface.

And in a single moment of utter fatigue and powerlessness, I surrendered to . . . . I don't even remember! It might have been a spoonful of peanut butter or a single lick of chocolate frosting or even the final bite of leftover French toast from Travis or Taylor's breakfast. Whatever it was, it was miniscule. It always starts that way. But what happened after the capitulation was anything but miniscule.

You know by now how these scenes play out. I eat something "bad." Regret inhabits me and starts to devour all the good parts of me like a cancer. The inner judge reports I've just committed a mortal sin, so I spiral into a whirlwind of punitive options for atonement. The sentence I must serve depends on the severity of the crime and comes in many shapes—a harder workout, a longer run, a crazy made-up diet. Sometimes the judge shows leniency and hands down a smaller sentence like just skipping one meal. But there is *always* a sentence.

This time the emotional devastation of the scene was much harsher however. I had come so far with exercise and motherhood and blood sugars. It had been years since I'd binged and then purged the old way—not years since restriction, just years since bingeing and following up with insulin omission. Bingeing had almost become history's misery by now. Body consciousness was still just as all-consuming and thinness was still just as important, but I had learned to "manage" these better with exercise, so if on a rare occasion of eating some unplanned temptation bothered my sense of progress, I simply worked it off, placing the iniquitous high sugar binge on the verge of extinction.

The higher the climb, the harder the fall. Whether it was that the spoonful of peanut butter or the single lick of frosting or the bite of French toast tasted that fantastic or caused that much regret, I can't say. But whether it was pleasure or guilt, or the toxic chemical reaction of pleasure *and* guilt, it caused me to pursue more of it. And more led to more led to more and more. . . . and before long, the ravenous glutton in me was unleashed once again.

If you've ever watched a monster movie, you know that when the monster is apprehended, once he finally escapes, he returns with a vengeance so strong that he will knock down buildings to retaliate. Nothing gets in the way of his retribution. There was a monster in me now, and he was bound and determined to destroy the city I had built. And that monster produced a sugar high so crippling that I was entirely incapable of parenting the two most precious gems of heaven that had ever fallen into my world. They were innocent and undeserving of a mother so horrible and selfish.

I called the school where Russ taught. I told him I was sick, but I didn't tell him why. And this devoted husband and loving father drove all the way home, collected his two-year-old twins, drove them to my mother-in-law's home, then drove back to school to fulfill his duties as a sixth grade math teacher. At the end of the day, he made the same stops in reverse and then arrived home where he very compassionately tended to his sick wife and played the dual roles of dad and mom to two energetic toddlers.

Speaking From Experience: Inspirations to Invite Healing

• **Child-Talk**

Is there a child in your life? She or he doesn't have to be your flesh and blood, but the child should be one that you love or at least care deeply about. Think about all the qualities of this child you adore so deeply—a smile, a giggle, the way she mispronounces a word or mixes up sixes and nines. What is unique about him or her? What is quirky or cute or so downright precious you could hug him to pieces? What hopes and dreams fill your head and your heart for this wonderful miniature individual who has barely begun to experience the world, this uncontaminated soul who is just beginning to create her own story and learn how that story fits uniquely into the bigger story of humanity? What can you say to cultivate the soil so that it embraces all the seeds of wonder that lie undiscovered in the footsteps ahead? What nurturing secrets can you share? Think about this child—not just in your mind; in your heart. Unleash your adoration, right now, in this moment. . . .

Now, this child—is you. Talk to her. See her. Recognize the wonderfulness in her, of her, about her—the wonderfulness that is here in this present moment, and also the wonderfulness that exists only in its potential state, in possibility.

• Phone-a-Friend

Next time you find yourself trapped at the mercy of the "mean-girl" inside your head, leave yourself a voicemail venting all the ugly things "she" is telling you about yourself. Don't hold back. Okay, I know; you feel a bit—um—silly. You'll get over it. Trust me. And if you just can't bring yourself to vocalize the harsh and hostile contents of your mind out loud, then email yourself instead. It's a bit less daunting.

When you feel fully expressed, put it aside. That's right. Don't listen to the voicemail or read the email right away. Click "send" and then forget you ever did this little exercise. Or even better, forget you ever had the ugly thoughts.

When everything feels good again and you know it will; it's the nature of the "ride," listen to the voicemail or read the email, but not as you. When you listen or read, it isn't your voice you hear; it's the voice of a good friend, your best friend, in fact. Be as fully present to her needs as you can be. How do you respond to "her"?

Write down your response and save it, whether you email it to yourself or just write it on notepaper and shove it underneath the socks in your dresser-drawer. Remember when you respond that this is the one person in the entire world you care most about.

Now, if that "mean-girl" voice should ever show up again, you are armed and ready for the "aha moment" of your life. Read your note or email. Believe every word! And know that *you* are your own best friend.

8

Verdict: Diabulimia

Diagnosis Number Two

Why do people assume that a person must be grotesquely underweight to have been afflicted with an eating disorder? Well, maybe not everyone assumes that, but I did, which is precisely the reason I was surprised when Dr. Brown referred me to an eating disorder specialist. Even if the numbers on my chart had not been boldly staring her in the face, couldn't she see with her own two eyes that I was by no means underweight? Yes, I found willpower to be one of life's major hurdles. Who didn't? There was no denying that placing thinness above virtue was perhaps a bit warped, but these traits described the majority of women in my world and no one accused *them* of having an eating disorder.

> **Anorexia** is an eating disorder characterized by refusal to maintain a healthy body weight and an obsessive fear of gaining weight. It is often coupled with a distorted self image.

So what, if my decisions were governed by the scale at times! So what, if I went a little overboard to fix a "wrong" on occasion! That meant I was human, not anorexic. I was levelheaded enough to know some of my methods of making things right again weren't ideal. But heck, we all make mistakes. It's not like I planned to screw up, not like I premeditated on it or anything. Most of my solutions were just quick fixes, nothing more than temporary and finite strategies: skip dinner—only for *this* week; double sessions at the gym—only for *one* month; no insulin—just for *tonight*. They were simply interim methodologies to facilitate a return to where I'd been before the transgression, a sort of indemnifying.

So how was I, now weighing a healthy 101 (*never* once in adulthood to dip underneath 92!) to buy into this anorexia diagnosis? I was a mere four pounds below the medical ideal for my five-foot-two-inch frame. Anorexics and bulimics were those skeletal figures you see in magazines or on talk shows with lifeless eyes, colorless skin, and bones protruding from beneath their oversized sweatshirts and baggy jeans. Clearly I was not one of *them*.

The truth is: not everyone who is skinny has an eating disorder, and not everyone with an eating disorder is skinny. It's not about the size of your body; it's not about the amount of food you eat or don't eat. It's about your *relationship* with the food; and it's about what *that* does to your relationship with your body.

Well . . . . maybe I wasn't like a typical anorexic on the outside, but on the inside, I had to admit, I fought the same war. The war where food had all the power, fat was a failing grade, and the bathroom scale was the report card that decided what you were worth on any given day. And just like those skeletal characters on the talk shows, I feared that failing grade and did anything necessary to escape it. *Anything*. Sometimes that "anything" happened to be sensible and healthy like ordering salad as a main course or taking the day's workout up a notch, but often it was preposterous or toxic—or possibly even life threatening. It didn't matter—not to the talk show people, and not to me—as long as we didn't fail. If you stood at the doorway of that failure, it didn't matter how you actually kept from crossing over, only that you did. Some did it with starvation. Some did it with regurgitation. Some did it with compulsive exercise. Some did it with diuretics. Some with laxatives. I did it with nearly all of them (except the laxatives). And I had an extra tool, my trump card—insulin omission (the single fringe benefit of having diabetes). It was the same war, the same obsession, just a different barricade keeping you on the "good" side of that doorway to fatness.

Diabulimia refers to an eating disorder in which people with Type 1 diabetes deliberately give themselves less insulin than they need, for the purpose of weight loss.

I always knew that my desperation to lose weight drove me to do things that weren't great for my body. I had never fooled myself into believing it was actually smart or healthy behavior. But I did it anyway, put my body in harm's way on purpose, for the sake of avoiding the failing grade. I was usually capable of functioning reasonably well in the midst of a *ketoacidosis* episode and I always seemed to bounce back. Okay, so maybe I'd have to someday face diabetic consequences like blindness or kidney disease or amputation. But that would be much later in life. Medical research was so accelerated and progressive these days, they'd come up with a cure for all complications of diabetes by the time I needed it—if I needed it. Heck, not everyone who smokes develops lung cancer! So yeah, I knew it was bad for my body, but maybe I never realized just how damaging it was for the rest of me. I was sick. I couldn't deny it another moment.

In 1971 I had been diagnosed with a diseased pancreas. Today, twenty-six years later, I was diagnosed with a diseased self-worth.

Allow Me to Introduce You to My Other Self

I don't remember the first time I met Sonya. She said it was when I was six months pregnant teaching step aerobics at the gym (using a towel, mind you, as a stand-in for my step). But I did not remember her. I think the only thing that registered for me during my pregnancy was my nausea and fatigue. I may not remember our first encounter, but I'll never forget *her*.

She was a large woman with a meltingly warm smile and a crazy sense of humor. She added life and laughter to every one of my classes she attended. She always stood in the same spot in the back right corner of the room mumbling things to herself and those around her, usually mocking her own inability to execute whatever instruction I happened to be demonstrating in the front of the studio. She would exaggerate her struggles with the moves and amplify her own labored breathing. Anyone standing in earshot would burst out in whirlwinds of uncontrollable laughter at her feigned self-deprecation. Whenever I was able to hear her self-jabbing over the music, I laughed too.

"Heave-ho!" bellowed straight from the bottom of her lungs during one of our Wednesday night classes as we simulated a rowing action with elasticized resistance gadgets known as exer-tubing. She became the class clown of my fitness classes.

If you're a person who frequents the gym scene at all, then you're most likely familiar with the stability ball. When these fitness tools were first introduced in most centers, they were predominantly blue. It does not take an enormously bawdy sense of humor to imagine the types of off beat comments this combination of "blue" and "ball" would occasionally elicit. Sonya was *that* member, the one with the comment. It wasn't even what she said that made her so funny. It was the way she got such a kick out of herself. You simply couldn't *not* laugh if Sonya was in the class.

Sonya approached me after class one day with a photo of herself.

"Since you don't remember me when we first met, I just wanted to show you what I *used* to look like." She placed the photo on the stereo cabinet. "This was a-hundred pounds ago!"

Wow. 100 pounds! This was not the same woman. She had come so far. How? I was suddenly in awe of this woman who brought such a treasured gift of laughter to my classes.

I came to learn that Sonya had a five-year-old son who was autistic. She did it for him, she explained. Well, she did it for herself, made herself healthy, so that she would be around for him. Sonya told me how much of an inspiration I had been to her back when I was pregnant. If I could "stand up there in front of class with twins in tow, green face and all, and persevere through that kind of stormy misery," she told me, then certainly the least she could do was to get herself healthy enough to stick around for her undeservingly challenged little boy. She also told me what an inspiration I was to her still, mother of twins, full-time job, and continued commitment to fit and healthy.

Sonya was motivated. She was also motivat*ing*. Knowing that I contributed to inspiring one hundred pounds worth of achievement for another human being was huge for me. I felt so . . . . significant. Sonya was one of those gym members who offered me a sense of professional triumph and credibility. She made me feel inspiring. And paradoxically it was this awareness of my ability to impact *others'* attitudes toward fitness that took me out of myself. It was empowering.

Sonya and I became friends. She was fun to be around, but she was more than fun. She was a wonderful person, a devoted mother, a caring hospice nurse, a loyal friend. Her smiles could melt glaciers. Her laugh could heal cancer. She was in love with three people: her husband, her son, and John Denver. But more than these, she was in love with life. And if you were one of the lucky ones to know her, she made you fall in love with life too. She was a woman with a large body and an even larger soul. And to my eyes, she was beautiful.

Sonya often asked my advice on how to "tone this" or "get rid of that." I gave her the patented answers my professional training had prepared me to give, and I tried to sound inspiring. On one occasion, Sonya asked me how to "find motivation." This particular question was a common one, but it caught me off guard coming from her. For me, Sonya personified motivation. She was motivation itself. *She* was the one who lost 100 pounds, not me. *She* was the expert, asking an amateur for advice on something she knew better than anyone.

But something about *this* question, coming from *this* woman, made me see myself with different eyes, eyes that weren't quite so—nearsighted. I realized in that moment who I had become, for her and for all the others who attended my classes day after day, week after week, year after year. I symbolized something important for them. I was struck with an eye-opening awareness of my real responsibility to not only talk the wellness talk, but to *be* what I represented—for them and for me. They did not see the fat person that lived inside me, the person that moved into my body the day I tried on that ugly green dress decades ago. They saw an icon of fitness, an example of health and wellbeing. I wanted to be the person they saw. I really wanted to *be* her.

I only knew Sonya for a few years. In July of 2001, she was diagnosed with a rare type of leukemia. Our gym sponsored an aerobicathon to raise funds to help defray childcare expenses for her autistic son. I and a few other instructors volunteered to lead it. It was a big success. In October, I attended a dinner dance fundraiser that Sonya's family and friends put together for the same cause. My table included a group of members from our usual Wednesday night class. One of the women took out her cell phone and called Sonya in her hospital room. It was the last time I would ever speak to her.

On Easter morning, 2002, Sonya died. At her wake—or rather, her self-titled "Celebration of Life" (which she had planned in great detail from her hospital bed)—they played a John Denver song. There were many of her loved ones who seemed to be slightly comforted by the idea that Sonya might now actually get a chance to meet him. Then they played a recording of Josh Groban's *To Where You Are*. It was a song I had introduced to Sonya during the cool-down stretch at the end of one of our Wednesday night fitness classes. On the following Friday morning I sang at Sonya's funeral. It was the only thing I could do for her now.

Every now and then during the course of one of my fitness classes, I call out an instruction like, "Okay, let's go grab the blue balls," and Sonya shows up in my head. Then she shows up in my sense of humor. She will always be very much alive there.

Speaking From Experience: Inspirations to Invite Healing

• Laughter

There is a hidden value in laughter that burrows deep inside the core of our overall wellbeing. The medical profession has come to recognize it as a highly useful instrument in supporting not only our mental wellness, but also our physical health. It reduces physical pain by releasing endorphins more potent than morphine, dissolves tension, stress, and anxiety that contribute to hypertension and heart disease, and increases oxygen in the blood which encourages healing and boosts the immune system. Laughter massages our bodies from the inside out, engaging all of our organs in a highly pleasurable and positive experience. It's great exercise for your abs too!

While this is all true, it sounds a bit too textbook and scientific for me. As a rule, genuine laughter isn't something that happens *on purpose*. Its usual way is to slip in through the side door and sneak up on you. Would we have it any other way?

• Where to Find It

So if laughter isn't really something we can "schedule" into our daily wellness routines, is there a way to create the conditions to get more of it on a regular basis? We could deliberately look for some naturally occurring humor in the everyday goings-on of our world. There's really no need to travel to the nearest comedy club or watch a favorite sitcom to pin it down. Life spontaneously presents us with humor all the time. It's built into everyday—if we let our guard down long enough to recognize it. We just have to be open to receive it and it will find us.

But there's a more effective way. Humor generally tends to have an easier time landing in the hearts of those who are willing to laugh at *themselves*. Simply letting go of any and all expectations we hold ourselves to, even if only temporarily, will help us to stop taking ourselves so seriously and will optimize the setting for laughter to happen.

• The Payoff
There is nothing that works faster to bring our minds and bodies into balance than a knee-slapping, floor-pounding belly-laugh. Humor lightens our loads, instills hope, and connects us to each other like nothing else. With such power to heal, renew, and replenish, the ability to laugh is a tremendous resource for overcoming insurmountable crises, rediscovering clarity, enriching our relationships, and supporting our physical and emotional health.

So go ahead and put yourself in the presence of those people who tickle the hell out of your insides. You know who they are. What are you waiting for?

9

Breaking Illness Open

The Rock

Triggers. If I could find a way to avoid them altogether, certainly I'd stand a chance to nail healing once and for all. Triggers were those cruel callous troublemakers that so effortlessly succeeded in pushing me over the edge right into the merciless claws of a binge. But what were they? Who were they? This was the topic of one of my sessions with Dr. Anderson, the psychologist I was now seeing at Joslin Clinic every week.

Identifying these villains was sure to be something of a lengthy drawn out investigation. Anything and everything could be a trigger. They were nondiscriminatory, known to attack from a different place every time. Fatigue. Boredom. Rejection. Disappointment. Self-importance or self-unimportance. Feeling empty or full or excited or anxious or lonely. All of it.

Dr. Anderson asked me to describe my last binge. I remembered it clearly. I even recognized the trigger's name: Stress. What had I been stressed about? Work, I think. (But it wasn't just about work. It was never just *about* anything.)

"Work is busy," I responded to Dr. Anderson. "Like all jobs, I suppose. The phones are nonstop. Our inboxes are overflowing. Then you get a call from a customer who is upset and you have to play the perpetual middle-man between the customer and the company."

"Then I go home where two tired hungry toddlers need some attention from their mom who they haven't seen all day. They deserve it and I want to give it. But if I do, dinner will be delayed and then they'll really be needy. And they can't understand. They're not supposed to. They're *two*!"

"In the meantime, I know I have a window of just one hour to give Travis and Taylor less than one-tenth of the attention they deserve, get dinner ready, and get myself out the door to teach a class at the gym." I recognized the familiar whiney voice now making its grand entrance past my lips. "*And* this leaves me zero time to review my choreography for the class I'm about to teach, which by the way, is expected to motivate a room of thirty people!"

(And zero time to fuel my body, which was about to execute a grueling workout!)

So where did the binge come in? Right after class. I poured myself a bowl of Kashi cereal. Fuel at last! It tasted fantastic. It tasted rewarding. But not rewarding enough to erase the stress of that day. So I poured another. And then another. And then another . . . . this time with some walnuts sprinkled over the top. And I didn't measure—any of it.

When my brain was finally beginning to catch up with my stomach, I started to add up all the calories I'd just devoured. One-hundred-sixty ugly calories per cup. *One* cup? I'd just inhaled at least *six!* And a whole handful of walnuts too! The math was just so cruel. And the guilt and regret were even crueler.

"You feel bad when the binge is over. What do you feel during it?"

"Pleasure. At least during the first bowl. What else should I feel?" Why was it suddenly necessary to consult her about feelings that belonged to me?

"Just pleasure?" she echoed.

"Mixed in with relief, I guess."

"What else can you tell me about it?"

"What do you want to know? The cereal tasted really good because I was depleted. *Physically* depleted. It started as a good thing. I know my body needed the food. The problem is I don't have a shut-off button inside."

But if it was only about replenishing energy, why didn't I stop when I was adequately restocked? What made me cross that line from pleasure to repugnance? What was this food-spell really about?

"So your body needed food and you listened to that. Good. But you also needed something you couldn't yet put your finger on. So some part of you decided to let the cereal take care of that need too. Did it?"

I thought for a second. It was a really good question. The obvious answer was no, but "no" didn't feel like the whole truth.

"Actually, I think it did work," I confessed, "but only for the thirty seconds each bite rolled around in my mouth."

She wrote something down and then looked at me as if I wasn't finished talking. I guess she was right: I wasn't finished.

"I suppose when life feels hard, using food feels, in the moment, like the only way to separate being me from everything that makes being me so hard," I began conjecturing. "For those thirty seconds, it's all about the food. Only about the Kashi . . . . or the sunflower seeds, or the chocolate frosting, or the Fritos . . . . or, or, or! Whatever is rolling around in my mouth is the only thing that matters; none of the hard stuff."

I recognized my chatterbox-self coming out and suddenly thought, 'Okay Maryjeanne. You should shut up now.'

"When the pleasure part stops being pleasurable, how do you feel?"

"You mean when I get full and when my blood sugar starts to go up, right?" She just sat there, her facial posture unchanged. "I feel sick. And filthy. Really grimy. Not just in my stomach, in my whole body. But I don't stop because I keep trying to get back what that first bite offered me—the bite that separated me from myself. It doesn't work though. I can't get it back."

"What do you feel when you realize you can't get it back?"

"Anger maybe. Or regret." But before the words were fully out of my mouth, something pulled them right back in. "No, hate. That's what I feel."

"Hate for what?"

"For me."

My chin was starting to quiver as I choked in the tears that were fighting to come out. She was already scribbling something down on the note pad that had been lying on her desk unnoticed for most of the session. She finished writing and then rejoined our conversation.

"Do you ever have a hard time forgiving people?" Dr. Anderson's question may have seemed random to some, but I was learning to recognize her lead-ins.

No. I considered myself an extremely forgiving person. "I'm sorry," were quick fix-it words for me. Nothing stayed broken in the presence of those words. Nothing. I did not hold grudges. I didn't even feel any grudge residue inside me once I'd heard those words—from someone else. Had I ever just tried to say those two fix-it words to *myself?* Could I forgive myself? That was what Dr. Anderson was asking me. And I heard her question, but I didn't yet have the honest answer.

Imagine holding on tightly to a rock; grasping it as if rightness itself depended upon your maintaining possession of it. Now let that rock represent un-forgiveness. Holding the rock makes you feel as though justice is possible, as though keeping it clenched tightly in your fist will make everything right somehow. If you are standing on a cliff holding that rock, could you open up your fingers and just let it drop into the water below? Just let go without any chance of retrieval?

Now, what if I tell you that this rock, this object that *looks* like your only chance to right a wrong, has been gouging the flesh of your palms and fingers all along, digging deeper and deeper into your skin the tighter you clench it? The longer you clasp your fingers around its sharp surface, the more injury it inflicts upon you. What if your only liberation from its harmfulness will come from opening your fingers and releasing that rock from your grip forever?

This is how I have come to look at forgiveness, how I have now come to see forgiveness, not just toward others, toward *myself*. Not an exonerating. Not an erasing. Not even a fix-it. A letting-go. But I still needed to learn how to let go of the rock; that it was the rock itself that caused the greatest damage.

Novocain

Food was not the enemy. It never was. It was pure emotional Novocain. A few more broken pieces of Hershey's chocolate; another spoonful of Ben and Jerry's; one more slice of ooey-gooey pizza. But Novocain always wears off. And when it does, you are left face-to-face with the raw pain it was designed to keep you from feeling. Fully exposed to its cruelty. And the pain of a binge's aftermath is compounded with more pain still—a physically ailing body that insists on violently betraying you, a deep-rooted ache entrenched in your soul caused by uncompromising shame and guilt. Guilt. That's the captain of the entire enemy camp. There is only one winner in a war against guilt: non-crime. *If* it's a crime, don't do it in the first place. Or go ahead and do it—because it's *not* a crime. It never was.

No, eating was not a criminal act. What was criminal was the way I allowed it to take possession of me, to control me. Rejection, stress, fatigue, loneliness, worthlessness—all distinct flavors of weakness; all vital pieces of the collective human experience; and all things that immobilized me in the face of food. So what were the things that made me turn to food as if it were the only thing that mattered? And what were the things that made me turn away from it as though it were Satan-incarnate? What made eating so evil and not eating so noble? What reason could I possibly have to keep eating when my body was screaming at me to stop? What was I looking for in that food? Did I think it would magically transform rejection into acceptance? Stress into peace? Friction into harmony? Fatigue into energy? Emptiness into fullness? What went on inside of me when the ravenous werewolf reemerged, frantically, recklessly hunting down its next mouthful? What made that next mouthful so utterly imperative? What did I *really* need from it that made it so life-or-death?

Love? Maybe that's what Dr. Anderson might suggest. I imagined the sound of her voice probing me now. Was that it? Was I looking for love? Ridiculous! Love was everywhere in my life—Russ, Travis, Taylor, the rest of my whole family, my friends, all the friends in my fitness classes—I was blessed with countless reservoirs of love in my life. Abiding love. Authentic love. Unconditional love. Selfless love. Even the love of laughter. Love stood dressed as a different creature on every corner of my world, and even if I was greedy for more, I certainly ought to be intelligent enough to understand that a snickerdoodle was entirely incapable of offering me love. I would undoubtedly need to set Dr. Anderson straight—if we were to ever have this conversation somewhere other than inside my head.

But the voice returned. I'm not sure if it was Dr. Anderson's voice or my own, but it was probing again, investigating the darkest corners of my subconscious. What about inside you, the voice asked? Look closely. What do you see there? There, in that space where love is supposed to be—the kind of love you are supposed to have for yourself? What do you see when you look in *that* space? I looked hard. I wanted to see it. Even expected to see it. It should have been there in plain view, right where I thought I left it . . . . but all I could find were judgments and supposed-to's.

Funny, how love can wrap itself all around you. You can bathe in it, stand beneath it, on top of it, smack-dab-in-the-center of it; but if it is not inside you—*for* you—it's nowhere. And that hurts.

Rattlesnakes

"Tell me about your relationship with your mother," Dr. Anderson invited in one of our sessions during the following weeks. "Are you close?"

Whoa . . . this was not a yes-no question. This was a whole new can of worms. No, not worms. Rattlesnakes. Were we *close?* It's a matter of timing and perspective. Growing up, there was no subject I couldn't bring up to my mother. Sex, drugs, love, God . . . . you name it. She invited intimate connection. Always. She actually impelled it at times. So yeah, I suppose the short answer would be: yes, we're close. But there were many words other than "close" to describe my relationship with my mom. Complicated. Challenging. Volatile. Deep. And if "close" made the list, so did "distant" (usually by my own hand). But I was here to talk about my issues with food and body image, not my relationship with my mother.

"We were very close when I was growing up," I answered, "but she is very needy and I think I push her away when I can't deal with her neediness. So I guess the honest answer is: close *and* distant."

"How is she needy?"

Another loaded question. She wasn't just needy in one way. She was needy in *every* way. She was needy because of who she was, and because of who she wasn't. She was an emotionally charged, overwhelmingly giving people-pleaser who could never receive enough approval to offset her feelings of inadequacy.

"She needs constant affirmation. It's annoying." Annoying? More like *impossible!*

"How does your dad respond to her neediness?"

"They're divorced. He could never give her enough love because she needs too much of it; because she doesn't love herself, even though she tries to make you *think* she does."

"That's an observation that takes a lot of insight." *Insight.* Etymologically—seeing inside. There certainly was a lot of *inside* stuff to see, so I suppose she was right. "Not loving herself enough must be a really sad way to live. It must hurt you to see that." She was right, but I wasn't exactly sure why. "What about you? Do you love yourself?"

No, I didn't. Not yet anyway. But at least I didn't pretend to. "I like some things about myself, but not everything. I just try to improve on the things I don't like."

"Like your weight?"

"Yes."

"Do you ever feel like you hate yourself?"

"Sometimes."

"When?" She was obviously leading me. I could see right through it. But I called her on it.

"I know what you're getting at. Yes, among other times, I hate myself when I've eaten something that I didn't plan on eating." There. I'm sure that was the answer she was trying to lead me to. Are you satisfied now, Dr. Anderson?

"Do you think that you're supposed to *plan* everything you do?"

"No, but when I'm trying to stick to a diet and I eat something I shouldn't, it's like breaking a promise."

"A promise you've made to yourself."

"Right."

"So you're seeing this broken promise as something that needs to be punished?"

I never thought of it as a punishment, but her word for it was a pretty good match for my general attitude toward cheating on a diet.

"I guess so. Not in a way that some parents would punish a child though. It's not like a punishment that's aimed to teach a lesson. It's more like something I need to do to make up for what I did wrong. To fix things and bring them back to the point where I was before screwing up."

"Like erasing your mistake?"

"Exactly."

"Do you think you're fat?"

Another question that was much more complicated than a yes-no answer would suggest.

"Honestly, no. I know I don't always handle food in healthy ways, but it's not exactly because I think I'm fat . . . . not really." I'd dropped seven more pounds and now weighed ninety-five. I was sensible enough to know that ninety-five pounds could only be considered "fat" if I were a toddler. "It's more my fear of *becoming* fat that drives me to overreact to a screw-up."

A little later in the conversation, she asked what I thought about my mom's relationship with food. Did I think my mom had issues too? Yes. Definitely. That was an absolute no-brainer. One lunch date with her would prove that truth to the world's biggest idiot. Here's how the beginning of a lunch date with my mom usually plays out . . . .

She apologetically breaks off the tiniest corner of bread from the breadbasket in the center of the table; guilt-waves radiate out of her almost visibly as she dares to go back for a second "corner," and then a third and a fourth . . . . You find yourself drawn into an inescapable trap of acute awareness of her bread consumption simply because she is trying so hard to make you (or herself) think she's *not* eating any of it. You fight hard to keep the angry voice inside you from blurting out, "Just take the whole piece, dammit!" Wouldn't it be so much less conspicuous (not to mention classier) to put an entire dinner roll on your bread-plate, eat what you would have eaten from the breadbasket in the center of the table anyway, then leave the uneaten portion to sit there until the waitress whisks it away? Ah, but then, she would not be able to tell herself, "I really didn't have a *whole* piece of bread, just a corner . . . . or so."

Did I think she had food issues too? You betcha!!! Funny thing is . . . . her apologetic and tentative approach toward food was hardly different from so many women with whom I'd lunched. This kind of bashful advance toward eating, especially in public, had become the cultural corset for womankind!

"Is your mom thin too?" *Thin?* Mom? Maybe I was painting the wrong picture . . . .

"No way. My mom has never *not* been on a diet." At five feet two inches, even when she had once weighed one hundred twenty-five pounds, she was still self-professed "fat." How could *I* then be expected to see anything other than "fat"? It was all *she* could see (whether the scale shared her opinion or not). And I was programmed to see it too. "So your mother thinks she's overweight then. Is she?"

"Yes." But she wasn't always overweight; she just made us both believe she was.

"You're repulsed by that?" What gave it away?

"Well, not repulsed," I responded impetuously. But I rethought the question and retracted my answer immediately. "Actually, I guess I am." I made it my personal objective to pull out every last crumb of authenticity I was capable of locating inside me during our sessions. But *this* conversation could not be straightforward and simple. Mom was a complex person and ours was a complex relationship.

"Is it all overweight people that repulse you, or just your mother?"

"No. Overweight people who are happy and self-confident don't repulse me a bit."

I thought about Sonya and how warm and beautiful her smile had been. Put her and my mother side-by-side and my mom would have appeared to be normal weight. But Sonya had been self-assured and content, with herself and with life. She celebrated what life had given her. What you really saw when you looked at her was her warmth and her sense of humor.

"Overweight people are like anyone else. Some are repulsive; some are attractive. Some are depressing to be around; others are a blast! I'm really not prejudiced against fat on *other* people. I've known many beautiful overweight people whose size I don't even see. I just won't stand for it on *me*. But my mother . . . . " I paused to attempt thoughtful articulation. "She *is* what I could become if I'm not careful. I'm not repulsed by her weight because of what it does to her *looks*. It's what it *stands for* that makes me resent it so much. Her weight is a consequence of giving up—on life and on herself. It's like she treats the most precious jewel in the Kingdom as if it came from a gumball machine!"

"The jewel. . . Is that a metaphor for herself or life?"

"Both I guess. She just doesn't value any of it—life or herself." But there were still so many more layers to peel off and wade through.

I guess you could say I was afraid of what my mom's fat symbolized, in the same way you might fear you'd inherited a parent's gene for breast cancer or Alzheimer's or Parkinson's disease. I was fearful of the possibility I might someday learn that I'd inherited my mom's "I-give-up!" gene. When there is something like this you perceive to run in the family, you do everything possible to arm yourself against it.

"She does it to herself," I continued. The rattlesnakes were all out now and they were completely free to have their way with me and my suppressions. "I understand willpower. We all can get weak. I'm no one to judge that. But with her, it's not just about willpower. It's that she lies to herself—about *everything*. She thinks it's been a successful day if she can convince herself she's eaten nothing but a hard-boiled egg all day. So I grew up believing it was a *good* thing to skip meals if you became desperate to lose a lot of weight fast. Not because she actually *did* it. Because she made it seem like a major victory if you *could*. And I tried it, but it's so difficult. Actually, it's almost impossible. And it doesn't work anyway. But she can actually convince herself that *she* can do it, not just once, but day after day after day after day—because naturally *she* has more determination, perseverance, and stamina than normal people. *She's* better than the rest of the world. *She's* invincible. *She's* superhuman! At least that's the bill of goods she's sold herself." Fury and disdain were beginning to boil together inside me. "But no one is supposed to be able to do what she *claims* she *is* doing. And it's a lie! I've heard her allege she's only eaten X, Y and Z today, right after secretly catching her in the act of shoving four thousand spoonfuls of macaroni and cheese into her mouth as she's cooking dinner . . . . for *'the boys.'* So yeah . . . . I guess I get a little repulsed."

Okay Maryjeanne, let's bring this conversation back to the present. Mom's not here in this room. Compose. Articulate. Stop exaggerating. Remember your commitment to truth and accuracy and stop letting your emotions and your fear do all the talking!

"But it's not because of her weight. It's because of the self-delusion that's so intricately sewn into her weight."

But if it was *her* self-delusion, why did it feel like it was all about *me?* If it didn't belong to me, how could it contaminate *my* fundamental beliefs about victory and failure? What on earth was I so afraid of?

Speaking From Experience:
Inspirations to Invite Healing

• **Metabolism Rut**

Enduring and effective weight management isn't about dieting. It never has been. It's not about *not* eating. It's about eating *more* of the foods that are satisfying and nourishing—to the body and to the self inside the body. All too often, the process of weight management is centered on scarcity instead of abundance. We're encouraged to enter into an arena where we play the almighty head-game of Deprivation Endurance. Though the rules of the game might be different each round, they are all equally irrational.

The body has a central intelligence that knows when we are overloading or under-loading it. And it will respond—in both cases. We know by now that when we eat more than we need our bodies store the excess as fat, but what about when we don't eat enough? How does the body respond? Does it suddenly begin to siphon excess energy from body fat stores in order to provide energy for daily activities? Quite the opposite. It slows down to preserve body fat. It senses the sudden deprivation and starts an emergency storage of every calorie consumed.

• **The Truth About Diets**

Year after year publishers continue to pump out diet books with real gusto, and guess what. Most of them work—and most of them fail. Why? Because they drench us with so many visions of our next meal that we forget life exists outside the imprisoning circle of this year's food rules.

Naturally we're eager to hear the newest research on food science. If the information turns out to be true, it's pregnant with promise. Therein lies the caveat—*if* it turns out to be true. We are confused. And we are desperately hungry for the truth.

• You Want "Rules" I Got 'em!

While I must confess that I haven't opened a single one of this year's diet books to learn what new earth-shattering secrets I might be missing, I'm confident that a little common sense will go a long way. So please allow me, once again, to help you wade through the plethora of confusion surrounding weight management and employ the K.I.S.S. principle (Keep it simple, stupid!) by following these seven simple rules:

1. Most importantly be as vigorously active as your life will allow you to be—doing what you love.

2. Eat food that looks the way the earth gave it to us as often as possible.

3. Drink water when you're thirsty not strictly to satisfy some arbitrary number of ounces.

4. Eat the food you enjoy and enjoy the food you eat. If you hate celery sticks, it absolutely will not serve you to eat them for lunch everyday—no matter how low they are in calories.

5. Fat is not a foe, but the kind you pour (like olive oil) will work better in your body than the kind you slice or spoon (like butter).

6. One final word about sugar—our planet gives us all kinds of sweetness. You might be surprised at how sweet veggies, whole grains and fruits taste once your taste buds get a break from sugar.

7. If your grandmother wouldn't recognize the ingredients, your body isn't likely to embrace them.

10

How Children Learn

My Mother's Legacy

I remember when Travis and Taylor were approaching the age of three, Russ and I decided to take a parenting course together. Needless to say, after our tempestuous six-year journey through IVF's, surgeries, and hormone shots, good parenting was pretty darned important to both of us and our circumstances convinced us it was unlikely we'd get another stab at it. Not to understate the obvious—that taking a class together was also a great excuse for a much-needed parents' night out.

Thankfully, quality parenting in today's world is understood to be more about raising adaptable self-confident individuals who welcome challenge and develop goals that are true to their own dreams than it is about producing perfect little cookie-cutter molds of Stepford children with impeccable etiquette and a promising future in medicine or law. So the relationship between praise and self-esteem was a hot topic during the few months we were enrolled in that course. How big a role should praise play in our childrearing? When to use it; when not to; how much; how little?

I remember the instructor cautioning us about giving children too much praise. She had said that, ironically, excessive praise is likely to contribute to *low* self-esteem. This perspective seemed to me to be a bit of an oxymoron, but she went on to explain that when we repeatedly praise children for their accomplishments, they grow to expect that pat on the back every time they do something good rather than learning to relish the pureness of their own intrinsic value. The alternative? Give them words to identify the good feelings they are already feeling inside for having done this good thing or achieved this challenging task. It made fantastic sense, but for me it was an entirely new methodology for fostering self-confidence. My mom had always been my biggest cheerleader. However, considering that it wouldn't be an overstatement to say that self-confidence and I did not have the most intimate relationship, I decided to open my thinking to the instructor's viewpoint.

Parents are our first glimpse of human relationship. They teach us important lessons about life, some deliberate and mindful, others entirely unaware and unintentional. My mom taught me many wonderful things. She taught me about optimism and teamwork, about the beauty in nature, and about the miracle of new life. She taught me about effort and practice and perseverance.

"If you really want to learn how to ride a two-wheeler, you have to work at it and keep working at it. It will happen. Practice makes perfect!"

Perfect. There's that word again. I heard it often. I wonder if every child took it as literally as I did.

No less frequently I also heard, "Nobody's perfect." But I wanted to be, so I'd just have to keep trying.

And my mom, with the grandest simplicity, taught me about the exhilaration of experiencing my mind and my soul soaring to new heights.

"How can God be everywhere at the same time?" the child me challenged often. The vastness of the notion of God always perplexed and stupefied me.

"Because God is like love," she would answer, confident and assuring. "You can't see love, but it's everywhere too. God is like that." Her answer satiated my unripe sense of the obscure.

My mom is a brilliant woman. She knows how to get inside the head of a child—especially *her* child—and respond in a way that impregnates a young mind with the richest nourishment. She understands things on a different plane than most people. I "caught" the depth bug from my mom early on. I learned to use it well. She truly nurtured my ability to grab onto the intangible. Depth has shown up in my life a lot—sometimes as a curse, sometimes as a blessing. And it would become indispensable in looking at the intricacies of my relationship with her.

Mom taught me so many wonderful things on purpose. I will always be grateful for the impact these things have had in shaping me. But some of the most powerful lessons came from the things she *didn't* intend to teach, the ones I learned by example.

Mom sought approval from others often—especially my dad. And I watched. I watched her light up when she received it, and I watched destitution overcome her when she didn't. I watched self-worth empty out of her like water from a bucket with a gaping hole. And I learned that worth is something you earned by being perfect enough—for someone *else*.

There is nothing that teaches you the value of something more than not having it. And like all moms, she wanted to provide for her children what I believe she was unable to own for herself. And so, that which she grew up craving so desperately, she tried her best to give to her children in abundance.

There could never be any doubt that my mom thought the world of her children; that she thought the world of me. There was more praise floating around that house than we could ever use up—so much in fact, that I didn't seem to develop the need for my own inner resource until much later in life. I was always amazing—in *her* eyes. Too amazing. But her eyes stopped mattering after a while because I figured out they could only see partial truths. Even more importantly, her eyes did not teach me to see myself the way she saw *me;* they taught me to see myself the way she saw *herself.*

I do not claim to understand the complexities of my mom's body image. I'm still learning about my own. But I know what I saw growing up.

"I gotta get rid of *these*," she would exasperatedly announce, grabbing a handful of flesh on each of her outer thighs. It was years before I would even begin to understand the notion of weight loss, but she believed it was so, and I believed her.

Her weight turned out to be just another one of those things for which she needed approval. The message I read from watching the way in which she directly linked food to her body was simple: Fat is not good; food is responsible for it; my dad would love her more if she had less of it. (Actually, whether or not my dad loved her curves never really mattered. When you can't nourish yourself from the inside, no amount of external approval is ever enough.) Children learn their most powerful lessons from the truths they witness, not the truths they are told. And so my mom had become my role model—of low self-esteem.

I think I saw Mom's sadness before I knew what I was looking at. And I studied her methods of trying to empty sadness from herself. I watched how she would turn to a half-eaten bag of potato chips to smother the sadness in her, and then act as if neither the sadness nor the potato chips ever existed. These were the strategies I'd witness over and over. These were the strategies I would make my own.

As adolescence would have it, I began to develop some body fat of my own. I was a good student of my mom's unintended teachings and I learned them well: Where body fat is, self-worth is *not*. And so the lack of self-worth that was hers now became mine. Maybe our pain was different, but to me it felt like it was the same. And I resented the sameness. Then I resented her. Though I appreciated having her diet expertise at my disposal when I needed it (or when I *thought* I needed it), I resented walking through the doorway to her world of perpetual diet obsession, but even more I resented standing there with *her*. She made it look like such a painful place to be.

Mothers intuitively strive for connection with their children, but I held on desperately to my separateness from her. I stopped sharing with her. Something about the prospect of allowing her to relate to *my* pain felt as though it would make us too alike in ways that I could not bear to be similar. Then it would stop being mine entirely. It would be all about her. So I instinctively shut her out, and though I battled intense levels of guilt over the rejection I was imposing upon her, my own emotional survival was at stake. It was not in my control. My intuition had taken over.

When I look through the lens of parenthood, the image on the other side of that lens isn't as blurry as it used to be. It shows me how natural it is to try and fix our own brokenness through parenting. Peeking through this lens I think I can see how Mom's overly generous affirmation of me and my sisters and brothers might possibly even have even been a sort of unconscious attempt to fix herself—or not. Either way, how could she have known that by filling my bucket of personal value from the outside, it would become harder for me to find the reservoir inside? How could she have known that I would pick up the same strategies of outsourcing that had left her empty? And how could she have known that I too might learn to equate my self-worth with the number on the bathroom scale?

Naturally, as parents, we aim to avoid making the same mistakes that we perceive our parents made. No doubt, I would make parenting mistakes too. But I was determined that one thing I would not pass onto Travis and Taylor was the legacy that was passed onto me: the dreadful habit of contracting out for an inside job. I would help them to find the treasures within them and not look to others to show them their greatness, even if it meant holding back a little on those occasions when I felt like singing their praises out loud from the top of the bleachers. As their mother, it was not my role to give them their personal worth. It was my role to help them discover and develop the tools to build it for themselves. The greatest good I could do for my children would be to learn to look at *myself* with different eyes. If I could somehow learn to find my own greatness, they would learn to find theirs.

Maybe this was the true legacy my mother had left me: the urgent necessity to develop the fortitude and strength to *not* need the external sanctioning that had become so imperative to her sense of self, the need to launch a full investigation of my own access to the greatness that already existed inside me.

How natural it can be to look outside ourselves for role models to emulate and admire when all the time we are already the example we seek. Self-doubt can cleverly conceal the wholeness inside that we crave, the same wholeness and confidence that we recognize so readily in those around us. Self-judgment can become more stifling than our perceived judgment by others. It can lead into an endless cycle of self-editing and an insatiable hunger for self-improvement.

I was an impressionable eyewitness to my mom's unquenchable craving for acceptance, approval and appreciation from my dad and others. She couldn't recognize it when it came because what she really needed was acceptance, approval, and appreciation from within her. I can only know this because now it was exactly what *I* needed to find too.

Affirmation from outside sources can't be trusted because it can be conditional. It can be withdrawn at any time. It is as nourishing to real self-worth as candy and bubblegum. But authentic self-acceptance is abiding. I wanted this for my mom. I needed it for me.

Speaking From Experience: Inspirations to Invite Healing

• Outsourcing
Does the way you feel about yourself on any given day seem tightly glued to some seemingly innocent external source—the bathroom scale, the full-length mirror hanging in your bedroom, a certain pair of jeans. A report card, performance evaluation, review or critique of something you've worked on, or some other form of verbal applause or criticism? If your honest answer is yes, stay with me.

• **Information versus *Relevant* Information**

First I'll address the elephant in the room: the bathroom scale. If your bathroom scale is properly calibrated, we can say it provides information that is true and accurate. But just because the information is true, does that make it relevant? What is the scale actually telling you? Is it declaring you a screaming success or pathetic loser?

I promise you the only *real* information that bathroom scale is capable of providing in any given moment is your body's relationship to gravity in the instant you're standing on it. That's it. Let me remind you, there's a whole lot more included in that number besides body fat. There are muscles, bones and fluids, not to mention a brain, heart, lungs, veins and nerves . . . . and not one of these valuable anatomical structures is weightless.

Let's face it—that bathroom scale is utterly unqualified to assess *you*. It offers no information of real value. The same holds true for the mirror, the jeans, and yes, even the opinions of others, which are always and exclusively reflections of what the observer is capable or incapable of perceiving. External sources will always lack credentials to perform the task of evaluating your worth. There will always be missing information in those "stories."

• **Call to Action**

I recognize that what I'm about to suggest may sound a bit extreme or drastic, but please hear me out. If the scale gives you zero essential information, why keep it around? If it daunts you, do away with it. You will survive, and even thrive without knowing that number.

So go ahead and be brave. Throw out the scale, take down the mirror, and start looking *inside* for the stuff that really makes you *you*, the stuff of substance that's been waiting there for you to discover it.

RENOVATION

11

Owning It

The Whole Pie

Cause—effect. Choice—consequence. Action—outcome. All naturally occurring inevitable responses that always become absolute realities. If A occurs, B results. Period. So, if I could isolate the cause of my eating disorder, it would stand to reason that I could expect to find freedom from it.

Did I think Mom was responsible? Let me put it like this: When you add sugar to berries, it turns them into a sweet fruity dessert. When you add that sugar to tomato sauce it reduces the acidity but does not make it taste sweet nor turn it into a dessert. The sugar is the constant; the berries and the sauce are the variables. I had five other siblings who were equally exposed to the influence of my mom's self-esteem. Not one of them developed an eating disorder, so how could Mom be responsible for mine? She was the constant. I was the variable.

I realize this may come as a surprise to you, but I honestly don't see my youth as one pathetic tapestry of dysfunction and pathology—actually, quite the opposite. For all of its impairment, it was far richer with love, laughter, and lessons. Sure, my relationship with Mom journeyed through its share of turbulence, but it was nonetheless nourishing and enriching and beautiful. It still is. You see one thing that took me a while to work out for myself is that Mom spent most of her youth in a childlike romance with the whole motherhood dance. To be honest, so did I, but at least I was an adult when I was invited to partake in that dance. She was only nineteen!

She couldn't have known all that the role would ask of her. And yet, she gave herself completely to it—to *me*—in spite of any emptiness that might have been scratching at her from the inside. Sure she had her baggage, but she was allowed to. Actually, she was supposed to. Who doesn't have a little rubble to work through? Maybe in the end, the rubble is even one of life's greatest gifts.

No, I genuinely did not blame Mom. I did for a while, but not anymore. I suppose when you grow up learning there's one person who fixes all the broken stuff in your world, you grow to depend on that, expect it. I guess it's natural that you'd blame her when you bump into something that can't be fixed. But I knew now that if I was to move forward into a space of true healing, it would be crucial to look honestly at all the pieces of the pie. My *perceptions* of Mom, my *relationship* with her—not Mom herself—produced just one slice of a very large pie.

What role did diabetes play? Despite my supposition that I'd invented the insulin-omission-purge, I'd learned that women with diabetes were actually almost three times more susceptible to eating disorders all along. So maybe it was fate. Certainly, the way in which the medical profession of the 1970's administered diabetic patient care and management led to some harsh restrictions for a typical egocentric ten-year-old. I remember feeling completely isolated from some of the greatest childhood flavor experiences— sauntering around a summer carnival holding an oversized puffy pink cloud of cotton candy; gorging myself with Nestle's crunch bars and Reese's peanut butter cups on Halloween night; freely ordering the chocolate shake with my McDonald's burger and fries. These were the kinds of seemingly benign pleasures I got to watch from the sidelines. Good ol' Mom. She really did her very best to fix my world for me. She would use all kinds of treat-imposters (like those cottage cheese and pineapple "sundaes") to make me feel like I wasn't missing out. She would try so hard to convince me that the imposters were even better than the real thing they were standing in for. Maybe she was really trying to convince both of us. It's only now, having stepped into motherhood too, that I can understand how hard it is to watch your baby missing out on something. But let me tell you, those "treats" ended up either really bad fakes, or I'd have to call them "cheats" anyway. Where's the fun in that? *Not everything that is broken can be fixed, Mom.*

My point is, as a pre-teen, having diabetes was just one more reason to feel different and deprived. What a perfect setting for this psychological arsenic to leech onto. After all, wasn't it diabetes itself that implanted this preoccupation with food in me in the first place? Management of the disease was all about food fixation—when to eat, what to eat, what not to eat, how much, how little. Obsession was practically encouraged. To eat without it would have been a luxury. Yet it was this very obsession with food that drove my pathological relationship with it. And let us not overlook the scientific fact that insulin stimulates appetite. (Kick me when I'm down, for God's sake!) Put diabetes inside a culture infatuated with skinny and campaigning against fat and you've got a perfect recipe for disaster.

Certainly I could not underestimate the significance of the fashion and beauty industry. Like most women of my time, I had grown up completely submerged in subliminal (and sometimes even overt) messages of the intimate relationship between beauty and thinness. All you have to do is pick up a Cosmo magazine with its airbrushed photographs of pencil-thin wafer-models, or watch reruns of Baywatch to see who our beauty heroes were. My already weakened and fragile preadolescent psyche was ill equipped to overrule these messages.

When I looked at the whole eating disorder pie, it could have been easy to point a finger at any one of these slices. But there was still one more piece, the largest one of all. . . .

At some point in life, it becomes necessary to take ownership of our choices. Regardless of where they had come from, regardless of how justifiable they may have been, *my* choices were essentially the ones that led me here. It would be easy to pass the buck, to trick myself into believing that the cause of my eating disorder was outside of me, but it wouldn't fix my brokenness. I knew I needed to somehow learn to rewire myself from the inside. I could make a contract with myself to immerse myself in all the "right" messages (now that I knew what the "wrong" ones looked like), marinate in them and absorb them until I would become so saturated with wholeness and healthy body image that there would be no possible way to drain them from a renewed, content, and self-accepting me. There was only one possibility for true healing, only one place to find it—inside me.

I knew it was going to be hard, but I was committed. Things were different now. I was different. I could start small, each day just by making one choice—not the choice to "be good today," but the choice to heal. Healing would probably ask something different of me each day—sometimes maybe even ask the impossible or the unreasonable—but I would listen to its requests and respond to them earnestly, no matter how difficult they would become.

A Kinetic Choice

The following is a journal selection from July 29, 1997. No further introduction is needed.

Enemy #1—ice cream! Today's trigger—a quart of mocha fudge almond, leftover from the kids' birthday party. I had forgotten it was still there, and it caught me off guard. But once that vision of forbidden decadence insisted itself upon me I couldn't push it out of my head. I had grown paralyzed with desire.

The truth, Maryjeanne. The *truth!* Look at yourself . . . really look! You look at others and you hear them tell you that they think they are fat too, but you don't see their fatness. You look at yourself and *feel* fat. But are you? Do you see it, or just feel it? Put yourself next to them and really look. And look again. With your eyes this time, not your self-esteem. You are not larger or fatter just because you *feel* it . . . and you have not in the last half hour just gained ten pounds just because your mind is telling you that you have. Wake up! You know this stuff! You have read enough nutrition books to fill the Grand Canyon, for God's sake! It takes 3500 calories to equal just *one* pound. *One!* You did not, just now, in thirty measly minutes of standing with your spoon to the more-than-half-eaten remains of a half-gallon of mocha fudge, consume ten times 3500 calories—35 THOUSAND calories! It is virtually impossible. Look at the facts. *See* the facts!

Stop giving this ice cream, this inanimate harmless mix of cream and sugar, so damn much power! You love science; look at it the way a scientist would look at it. See it not as the enemy or as a force greater than life. Look at it for what it *is*. It's ICE CREAM, not a crime! Look at the reality. It is nothing more than fuel, fuel for the body. Your body. What is your body really worth anyway? It's nothing more than a package that houses the substance of you, the mind and the soul of you. And if this ice cream is nothing more than some form of fuel, then it is energy. And energy is a good thing, a necessary thing. It's the reason this body continues to survive. And so what if you take in *too much* energy. What's really the worst that could happen? Your extremely proficient body stores it up for you to use later. Yes, it is called *body fat,* but don't turn that body fat—that clever manifestation of the human body's efficiency—into a tool to decide what you're worth. It's nothing more than stored energy. Energy to be used!!!

Can you really erase something you've done? Really un-eat a piece of fuel that you already swallowed? No … you can purge it but you cannot erase the occurrence of having eaten it … so now, that fuel is *in* there. In your body. And you have a choice.

You can leave it in there, to do its thing, to give you that energy when you *do* need it. Even if you don't need it now, you might need it later. Or (here's a bit of ground-breaking rocket science for you) you could *make sure* that you *do* need it later. And it will be there, waiting to be used up.

Or you could purge it . . . get rid of it. You could stick your finger down your throat and hope that every single fat and sugar gram makes it back out through the same doorway through which it entered.

Or . . . you could . . . skip your insulin again . . . let your body get sick . . . again. Then you will prevent that energy from coming in and attaching itself to your thighs or your waistline. But you will also prevent your body from absorbing essential nutrients. And you will feel just awful. Because you will be sick! Because you *are* sick. *SICK!* And your sickness has left you broken. You have a disease. Not just a disease of the body. You have a disease of body *image*, and you have a diseased self-esteem!

So—what is your choice anyway? Are you going to keep giving food all that power? Why don't you get real! Look at yourself! Has your size or appearance changed since you looked in the mirror an hour ago? Have *you* changed—*really?* Just because you ate that ice cream? You *feel* like you have, but look at the facts! Look with the eyes of the fitness guru you've chosen to be. *LOOK!* Don't decide what you see before you look. Open your mind!!! Look to *see*, not to confirm your preconceived fantasy of how fat you are. And now receive . . . the *truth!*

What do you want to do about that ice cream now? Do you still want to get rid of it?

Yes. I wanted to. But I didn't. I spoke firmly to myself. I spoke compassionately to myself. And I spoke sense to myself.

Tomorrow maybe I could use up just a few of those extra calories from that ice cream. And the next day, maybe a few more. It wouldn't take too long, just a couple of days. A couple of days to use up a few more calories than I might have expended if I'd never seen that leftover ice cream. What's a few days? I could wait that long for this ice cream to become a piece of my private history. Let it just be stored energy for now. It won't turn into body fat unless I stop using up energy. It'll be okay. I knew that I had won today's battle.

Chasing Perfect

We learn when we're young that pursuing our dreams and taking control of our destiny is a good thing, an admirable thing. But what if the dreams themselves are toxic? What if their shape has been twisted or warped? What if they disagree with Nature's decisions? How much control over our destiny is too much?

I had grown attached to a vision of a counterfeit self, a self that couldn't possibly exist, because the closer I got to the vision, the further away it moved from me. In reaching for a better me, the real me always disappeared into an empty promise.

Two pounds less this week . . . . a new and improved me!

Two more next week . . . . even better!

Don't stop.

You aren't there yet.

There is still a little pocket of fat over here. . . .

and there. . . .

keep going. . . .

someday you'll get there. . . .

Where?

To *perfect.*

But when? How many times do you need to step through better before you get to perfect? How many times do you need to step through better before you get to *good enough?*

I had robbed myself of so many real moments trying to arrive. Moments. *They* were the real thing. Ordinary, extraordinary, hilarious, rich, triumphant or even lonely—every single one of them with its own something real to offer. And I had let so many get away, all for the sake of a few more pounds, a few inches closer—to "perfect."

Maybe sometimes it's best not to dream, not to pursue, not to control. Maybe sometimes it's just better to trust; to let life decide for you; and then to embrace what it has given you—even if you don't agree with its decision.

I wasn't sure I'd ever entirely stop caring about my weight, no matter how unworthy I would finally come to recognize that pursuit to be. But I did know that I somehow needed to learn to stop living so attached to every last detail of this phony me I'd been chasing. Maybe I would never be perfect—whatever that meant—but I was already good enough. I had always been. We all are. We are Nature's finest and most complex art—hearts and lungs and organs and muscles and bones, unceasingly engaged in a well rehearsed, gracefully choreographed dance; minds and souls integrated, forever connecting the obscure puzzle pieces of life's biggest questions.

But I still needed to learn how to trust Nature's intelligence. If I did my part, Nature would reward me somehow. Maybe not the way I once would have wished to be rewarded, but it would reward me. For today anyway, I would make a choice. Not a choice of action. A choice of *non*-action. A choice of acceptance and trust. Nature had a lot to tell me. It was time for me to listen.

Virtual Deathbed

I know this is going to sound a bit morbid, but please indulge me for a few pages. If you really want to know how vitally important something is, just imagine yourself on your deathbed. Go ahead. Pick something—something enormously, fundamentally and intimately important. Create a space in your mind to bring yourself to those last few breaths of life, that final moment. Are you there yet? Now retrieve that vision of "important." How does it look—from *here?*

This is exactly where I took myself to honestly examine my values and stare down my warped obsession with my body's "flaws." But it wasn't only about the pathology of my body image; I looked at everything—everything that seemed like a big deal at one time or another. I wouldn't exactly call it an out-of-body experience, but some things really looked a lot different from this place.

How imperative had it really been to land that account, or get that promotion, or those shoes, that part in the play, or that next level on the fitness ladder? How earth-shatteringly catastrophic had those extra five hundred calories really been? Or those five minutes late to work, or that flat tire, or that petty misunderstanding, or the mushy overcooked asparagus that ruined dinner, or that bad hair day, or the escalating gas prices, or that lost wallet (stuffed with $200 cash!)? I looked at everything. *Everything*. The self-made ordeals, the mountains *and* the molehills, the triumphs and the failures; all the things that once tricked me into thinking that they mattered more than they really did. It had all been so uncompromisingly *important.*

Then I looked at my futile mission to find "perfect." All the inner debates about food and weight; the triumphs of a ten-pound weight loss and the punitive self-hate of a binge's aftermath; all the delegating of self-worth to the size of my blue jeans, the measurement of my waist, the unpremeditated samplings of chocolate chip cookie batter, the number on the scale; all the time spent chasing outcomes and punishing failures. What had it all done for me? What had I really gained? What had I really lost? How important was any of it—from this imagined place of near-death?

For the next moment of this daydream, I stood in my own stillness and watched truth impregnate silence. And then, as if seeing some unfathomable biblical miracle never before witnessed, I watched as the silence spoke louder than thunder. It said that not one of these had ever been even a little important. It told me the number on the bathroom scale said nothing about the life I got to live; nothing about the lives that had intersected mine; nothing about *me.* Whether it represented five, or ten, or even *fifty* pounds of subcutaneous flesh that embodied the stuff of me that made me me, it was meaningless in the end.

The fat I carried (or didn't carry) on my body had zero relevance to all the stuff I carried inside my heart—those rare moments of pure connectedness with another human being—talking with Russ during one of our long runs through the hilly farms of Causeway Street or on a Caribbean beach walk, a five-minute call with my sister Therese (that somehow always ended up lasting over an hour); my extraordinary children, now young adults—Travis and his willfulness, his wit, and the secret tenderness he keeps safeguarded inside, Taylor and her genuine compassion, her intuitive wisdom, and her utterly infectious giggle; my love for music, the outdoors, children, autumn foliage; all of those unexpected "mountaintop moments" of life; the honor and privilege of existing on this planet as one small part of an exquisite web of humanity and grace.

Fat was ignorant about that place in the center of my soul where love, gratitude, fervor, empathy, and even raw vulnerability all overlap. That place was precious, sacred. Whatever shape my body decided to take on at any time, the shape itself was blind, deaf and dumb to the real gifts I held inside me. Whatever value the artificial authority of my weight pretended to have at life's pit stops, here on this made-up deathbed, it could no longer hold me hostage.

This morose fantasyland I had dreamed up on purpose awakened me in a way I don't think I'd ever before been awake. Life had to be more than an endless search for thin. It had to be more than an endless search for perfect. Maybe . . . . "perfect" was already here. Maybe it always had been.

And it was here in this space, tightly sandwiched right between fear and fortitude, looking deep into the eyes of choice, that life, as I knew it, changed. I was ready. Ready to finally let go of something I'd been gripping so tightly it had blinded me for most of my years; ready to let the lie at last move out of my way; ready to stop buying every single word that bathroom scale kept trying to sell me about my personal worth.

Looking around at the new world I was already standing in, I exhaled. Could this be happening for real? Could it finally just stop mattering if I happened to eat a few more calories than I planned to? I tell you, this was truly one of those bigger-than-life "Oprah Light Bulb Moments," and I breathed it in as if it were the very first time I'd tasted pure oxygen.

But in less than a nanosecond, a fierce new awareness abruptly overpowered my newly discovered tranquil surrender, and knocked me down like a fast strike in a bowling game. It was the obtrusive awakening to the reality of wasted moments—moments shattered by my own hand, traded in for skinny-mania. What a miserable waste! Had I actually squandered away such gems reaching for something that had absolutely zero value? All the counting and measuring, the sacrifice, deprivation and commitment—for what! What a meaningless, sorry, pitiful misuse of life!

Or was it?

There's no denying that I turned to rigorous workouts for all the wrong reasons at first. Okay, so my unrelenting pledges to two-hour boot camps, eight-mile runs, and grueling weightlifting sessions may have originated with taco pie binges and frenzied pizza sprees, but did that have to mean that the workouts themselves were good for nothing? If you added up all my lifetime hours spent in The Cardio Zone, they were certain to have *some* redeeming value. Okay, so warding off cardiovascular disease, reducing my risk of cancer, and enhancing longevity may not have been my *reason* for being a workout-aholic, but I still got to reap all the benefits, no matter why I started. And certainly one could not overlook exercise's impact on preventing the foreboding complications of diabetes: retinopathy or blindness, neuropathy, foot amputations, and kidney disease, among others. If you put it in these terms, you could actually say that my obsession for thin and perfect turned out to be somewhat of an unsung hero—even if it did creep in through the side door.

Maybe it was time for me to look more multi-dimensionally, not just at this muddled relationship between food and body image, but at all of life's hurdles. The word "hurdle" after all is really just a synonym for teacher, right? Life gives us hurdles so that we learn important lessons. Sure, they're hard, but only as hard as we need them to be in order to learn what they showed up to teach us. If you don't learn the lesson at first, you keep trying. You succeed a little, and you fail a lot. The failures teach you things. And the things they teach you become links in a long chain of earned wisdom, necessary stepping-stones that connect you from where you were to where you are. And everything along the way, including the hard stuff—no, *especially* the hard stuff—evolves us somehow. Pain can in fact be the finger that points the way to the next destination.

So where was this new destination? What was so invaluable about having lived all of my youth pitting food against my body? Maybe this God-awful food-war was life's most effectual instrument for the *real* work that needed to be done—you know, the deeper lesson—the right tool for the right job. Maybe it was paradoxically the very darkness that allowed me to see the light of true Selfhood inside me in its most authentic form—the poverty that made me rich.

You must have figured out by now I'm a huge fan of metaphors. I often refer to life's obstacles as roadblocks or hurdles. (I know—overused metaphors grow pretty trite after a while.) A few years ago I heard a new analogy for life's hardships that I still like: "brick walls." What's so different about this one? Brick walls are the result of cumulative layering of brick and cement. They are not simply freestanding inconveniently positioned obstructions to progress.

The person I heard use this metaphor for life's struggles was dying of cancer. He didn't have to imagine living in the virtual deathbed; he was right then living in the center of its cruel reality.

Just before he died he said that the brick walls in our lives are here for a reason. It was a simple statement, but it felt incredibly powerful when I heard it and I agreed instantaneously. The brick walls always have something to teach us.

Life had given me diabetes. Diabetes had paired up with messages from all around me and constructed a "brick wall" layered with self-imposed limits and expectations of a fictional perfection. But I was beginning to break down that wall. Not in a single explosive attack though. It wouldn't work that way. Maybe you could knock down some walls that way, but not this one. This wall needed to be dismantled carefully, brick by brick, one layer at a time.

Okay, so maybe I didn't create all the bricks. Maybe I didn't choose the wall. But I was the one who had made the choices that cemented the bricks together. And I would have to be the one to break them apart. I had to admit, that here in this made-up final chapter of life, the "brick wall" itself had actually become one of my greatest teachers.

Speaking From Experience: Inspirations to Invite Healing

• The Quick-Fix Dilemma
At this point there can be no question about where I stand on the topic of diets and I think you'll agree I've made a pretty good case against them. I've offered you several compelling reasons why dieting doesn't succeed long term. In the end you will be your own jury.

Somewhere in the same camp as the futility of diets is a similar truth. To achieve *enduring* fat loss through diabetic *ketoacidocis* is irrefutably not possible. While I won't deny that for a diabetic body, fat loss is indeed achievable through overindulging in obscenely over-abundant amounts of food while simultaneously denying the body access to that food, fat loss accomplished this way is both potentially fatal and always temporary.

The body is designed to protect itself. When its wellbeing and functionality is threatened, its team of interrelated systems and structures goes full throttle into rescue mode with one mission—self-preservation. It will either succeed or it won't.

• Mortality
Recently as I was doing some research in preparation for a talk I was to give for parents of children with diabetes, I stumbled upon a few blaring statistics. The mortality rate for diabetes alone is 2.5% annually. The mortality rate for anorexia nervosa is 6.5% annually. It would stand to reason then, that the mortality rate of the combination would obviously fall at some greater statistic. But in reading on I was amazed to learn the mortality rate of Diabulimia is a whopping 34.8% annually!

I suppose there's no way to really know if learning this statistic sooner would have made an impact in abbreviating my illness, but I do know for certain that placing matters in terms of life-and-death possesses a unique power to transform morals, ideals, and philosophies.

• *Your* **Trip to the Virtual Deathbed**
Now that you've taken a trip to my Virtual Deathbed, I invite you once again to create your own. This exercise can be as involved or as brief as you want. Clarity, like balance, is in constant motion but somehow a short trip to the Virtual Deathbed has a way of transporting you back to where the waters are clear and illuminating the things that matter.

Once again, retrieve that vision of all the stuff that really counts, you know the critically important stuff. Imagine all of these things filling a large bucket and write a list of the items in your bucket. Look at each item on the list individually, asking yourself the same question for each one. Does it really belong in the bucket? Are there any items you might consider removing? What might you consider adding? View the list periodically and journal about the changes you notice. Observe how the bucket evolves over time.

12

Reshaping Tomorrow

Bridges, Backs, and Artwork

I'm not exactly sure how old Taylor was—maybe seven or eight—when she began to notice some of the wrong things about her mom, but I'm very sure it scared the hell out of me. It completely took me off guard. Naturally, having a daughter, I needed to anticipate crossing some of these types of bridges—eventually. Life had been slowly preparing me for them. But the day Taylor stood in my room with me as I freshened up to go out to teach one of my fitness classes, I was certain life had made a mistake. Her observations exceeded both my readiness and her age. But I knew there would be many more bridges ahead like this one to cross. And I knew I needed to be ready for them.

I was wearing a pink spandex sports-bra and a pair of fitness shorts. As I grabbed my Nike hoodie and tossed it over my shoulders, Taylor's words were chilling.

"Mom, I want a boney back like you."

My inner response to her unfiltered observations was twofold, simultaneously authentic and opposite. Their duality told me that there were still a few places left on this healing roadmap I had not yet visited.

On one side, a little girl narcissism reawakened inside me and I grew obediently exalted at the recognition of Taylor's uncensored remarks. They were innocent and judge-free observations, but I had spent a lifetime aspiring to a "boney" *anything,* and it was difficult to not feel affirmed, validated, approved of. After all, who doesn't know that the voice of a child always speaks the truest truth? Kids tell it like it is. They say what they mean and mean what they say. So if a boney back is what Taylor saw, I had no right to hold onto old baggage that said otherwise.

But it was the voice that came from another place that ultimately prevailed.

A boney back? Who notices a *back?* This was not supposed to happen. At least not yet. She was not supposed to notice things like this. And she was *not* supposed to care. I had done so much work inside to shield her from this sort of damaging body dissection. I had been so careful!

"I think you might be seeing *muscles,* honey. Not bones." I composed my response to sound as cavalier and matter-of-fact as possible.

"Well I like it," she insisted. "How can I get my back to look like that?"

The Question. I remember it well. I had asked it daily. Hourly! Maybe not about the back per se, but it was the same question. Even if I didn't vocalize it, The Question was always there. It was integral to every molecule of my existence. "How can I get my . . . to look like that?"

What could I say to my precious beautiful child to cultivate the soil of rescue—to prevent her from setting one foot into the zone of Perfection Hell? I didn't want her to spend one minute there! She didn't deserve it. No one does. But please, God. Not *her.*

"It comes from many, many years of hard exercise" was the best I could come up with.

You know what happens, Maryjeanne, when children hear untruths or twisted truths, I reminded myself. They see the truth eventually anyway. They need truth. Maybe not all at once, but they need truth, not lies. So offer it in small installments. Not too much. Not too little. Let Taylor's questions guide you to give the answer she needs to hear, the answer *you* once needed to hear. Don't just hear her words. Hear her curiosity. Fuel her. Nourish her. Shape her sense of her body.

"When muscles get stronger they stick out more and you can see some of the smaller sections of them more clearly." Whew! Where did that come from? Maybe life didn't make a mistake after all. Maybe the almighty book of parent dos and don'ts would say I was actually handling this okay.

"Will you show me some exercises to do?"

"Sure. But remember you're a child and children's muscles take many years to fully develop."

"I know." But Taylor's thirst for a predictable outcome was as naïve as her optimism. "Do you think if I do the exercises you show me my back will look like yours when I'm a grown-up?"

I thought for a second. I was sure she interpreted my pause to mean I was considering what exercises to show her, but the reality is I needed a moment to map out the healthiest route for this dialog to take.

"I don't really think anyone can know exactly what a child's body will look like when she grows up," I finally confessed with resolve. "But here's what I do know: If you decide you want to exercise, you'll grow strong and healthy. Then your back—*and* the rest of your body—will reward you in ways you can't begin to imagine. And if you put all that exercise together with healthy eating, you will look exactly the way you are meant to look, the way God wants you to look." In those days Taylor happened to be especially inquisitive about God, so I was confident in her ripeness for where I had finally decided to take this conversation. "There is no greater artist than God," I continued. "And *we* are his best art project. One of our most important jobs in life is to take our very best care of God's finest art."

As the words left my mouth, I knew that I was not only talking to Taylor.

Reflections of a Box

I guess I've always been a fan of presentation. Appearances have always mattered, even when I pretend they don't. I was practically born with a lifetime subscription to the fashion ruling, "accessories make the outfit." When I entertain, I have a history of being a stickler about garnishes and visually attractive menus with a balanced color palate, not to mention color-coordinated table linens. And when I'm the one who gets to choose the restaurant for dinner, ambiance has tended to bias my selection more than any other criteria. I am predisposed to favor the elegance of wine over beer (with the exception of beer served in a *fluted* glass), but I prefer cabernet served in oversized bubble-shaped wine glasses and chardonnay in the tall pear-shaped ones. (I'll pass, thank you anyway, if you dare to offer either to me in a *plastic* cup.) When I bring a gift to a baby shower or present you with a Christmas gift, my excitement steps up a few notches when it's wrapped in one of those attractive gift-wrap ensembles with coordinating embellishments.

Yes, I've always been one of *those* people—but not quite so much anymore.

Taylor was nearing the end of her grade school years. I lay down next to her in her bed, like I usually did during those years, and I rubbed her back to help her wind down for bedtime. Like I often did during this ritual of daily pause, I offered my daughter a bedtime "snack" of affirmation.

"You have such nice smooth skin," I commented.

"I hope I don't get a pimply back when I'm a teenager," she blurted out, slightly breaking the tranquil rhythm I was aiming to establish for bedtime. "I think it looks gross."

Though the disparaging statement seemed extremely un-Taylor-like, I exonerated her momentary shallowness and rationalized that she had been spending a lot of time recently flipping through teen magazines notorious for preying on a young girl's desire for a plastic kind of attractiveness. It was an instantly identifiable teaching moment for me, the kind parents look for, and a shiny golden opportunity I didn't want to miss. I interpreted her impromptu remark as an immediate call to purposeful parenting.

"What if you had two boxes in front of you," I began, "one box wrapped in bright colored paper and a matching bow with some really cute ornaments and the other wrapped in plain paper—the color of a Roche Bros. shopping bag—no bow, no frills. Which one would you pick?"

"The colorful one, wouldn't you?"

"Yes," I had to admit, "I probably would. I guess it might be a little easier to imagine the pretty package held a better present inside." I paused for a minute to search her eyes for a hint of recognition of where I might be leading her. "But what if the better gift happened to be inside the plain box instead?" I continued. I could see her trouble-shooting naïve mind beginning to work through a way to ensure a personal victory either way. "It's kind of the same with people I think. Sometimes we forget that the real gift is inside, especially when the "box" isn't particularly good-looking. Don't you think we might miss out on some pretty awesome stuff this way?"

I continued to rub her back, feeling proud of myself for recognizing this subtle invitation to impart an important lesson to my preadolescent daughter at such an impressionable time in her life. I hoped I was planting a seed that would someday blossom into how she would come to see herself.

"Who says you can't pick both?" she said after a long, thoughtful silence.

And in an instant, my message felt surprisingly less poignant. She had clearly taken my point even further than where I had intended her to take it. The moral of my made-up scenario had just been one-upped by the one who was supposed to learn from it. By overlooking the possibility of something wonderful within the pretty package, and acknowledging that potential only inside the plain box, I had failed to recognize that both packages promised value. Good for her, I thought! She had seen that the packaging itself had zero relevance to its contents. So why settle for just one if neither is guaranteed comparative excellence?

Did my own affinity for eye-catching packaging make me shallow? Did it mean that I was oblivious to the fact that there could be a true gem inside all packages? Of course not. It just meant that I loved a pretty box. The box did not *define* its contents. It just *contained* it.

The human body was a box of sorts too, I thought. Maybe I'd once overlooked that. Sometimes my "box" might not have been the shape I wanted it to be. Sometimes I'd wished it had come with prettier wrapping or a different color bow or frillier ornamentation (or a tinier waist or longer legs!), but it was still just a box. And it was *my* box, the only one I would ever have. Art. *God's* art. Who the hell did I think I was to try to improve upon *that?* I was not the box. I *am* not the box. I am what's *in* the box.

Taylor knew what her mother had forgotten: You have to unwrap the gift and *open* the box in order to know what's inside. Did I really *not* know that?

Trans-generational Repair

As my first role model, my mom was the one who had represented for me what women were, in every sense. So naturally, as a little girl, I naively accepted that all women were *supposed* to care that much about their weight, that our success and our worth was accurately measured in terms of how little we ate or how little we weighed. That's the message I received as a child. Whether or not her claims were true was entirely irrelevant. Her frequent boasting about eating next to nothing all day told me that achieving that feat was nothing short of a small victory. Victories enlarge your self-worth. It's not surprising then that I grew to equate my value, at least partially, to willpower and weight loss.

Fast forward to a more recent time. My sister Therese and her family were visiting from New York. A visit from Therese is a treasured event for the entire family, so I invited Mom to join us after dinner and sit by the fire to enjoy time with all of us. One of the very first things out of my mom's mouth as she plopped herself on the couch in our family room was the familiar boast accompanied by that all-too-familiar bravado.

"I lost twelve pounds this week!"

Isn't it funny how just a few wrong words from the wrong person have this uncanny ability to awaken the inner adolescent? I was instantaneously triggered. Twelve pounds? Really? In just one week? Not seeing it, Mom. Funny—in my world, the only possibility achieving such extreme results would put you in the hospital. My teeth were beginning to grind.

"Well *that's* healthy," I blurted out, exploding with sarcasm. "Certainly not something *I'd* be bragging about." Someone had to model sensibility for all the little girls in the room. I pursed my lips firmly to prevent further hurtful derision from slipping out.

I refused to pretend anymore, but more importantly, I did not want these children—*her* granddaughters—these innocent sponges ranging in age from eight to fourteen, to presume for one nanosecond that there could possibly be anything virtuous about the corrosive link she still created between weight loss and self-worth. I hated that Taylor and her cousins had to see that level of importance placed on a twelve-pound weight loss or *any* weight loss.

Taylor witnessed the entire exchange and she later reprimanded me for my callousness. "Mom," she started, "I think you made Nana feel bad. Even if she didn't really lose twelve pounds, why do you have to make her feel bad? Obviously she *wants* to lose weight. Can't you just keep that stuff in your head?"

Taylor had seen, and she had heard. And she would have been right. But she was not around for the beginning of the story. She was incapable of seeing the history of rigorous work I had already done to flush out all the toxins of childhood. And she didn't know how painfully hard I had already worked to recover from the damage of its influence, how difficult that war within me had been, how difficult it was for me still to prevent that inner war from returning, or how triumphant it was for me now to have loosened its imprisoning grip.

Taylor did not know because I had shielded her, or at least I'd hoped to. As far as she knew, this kind of autoimmune suppressed self-destructive thinking was just juicy material for her fiction novels. And it only plagued other families, not ours. Not ever. I'd made damn sure of that.

How many times I had climbed on my soapbox to preach my mind-body clichés.

"Make healthy choices *most* of the time, not *all* of the time."

"Exercise should be fun!"

"Take care of your body and you'll have the one that God intended you to have."

"Inner beauty is what really matters."

But she couldn't know where my words had come from. To her, they were simply emblematic mother's platitudes that all moms say to their children. She didn't know that I'd earned every bit of these wise words the hard way. All she knew at that moment was that her mom was being mean to her Nana. And her Nana, (who hadn't yet broken free from the food-body chains of our time) was now clearly injured by *my* insensitivity.

Hiding our weakness and pain from our children won't teach them strength. Children learn by seeing what is real. They learn by the example of our own resilience, our own healed injuries. By allowing them to witness our resourcefulness in developing strategies for coping with difficulty, they learn how to draw on their own strengths and build on their own resilience.

And so, the following day I shared with my daughter. I shared the history of my epic struggle with body image; I let her inside to where those hurtful words to her Nana had come from. And then, the very same night I did something very difficult, and very powerful—for me. I called Mom. And I let *her* in too. And then I apologized for the hurtfulness of my words. But she had already known where they originated. And she had already forgiven me.

I wished I had been capable of a different response to Mom the day of that visit. But just as Taylor had missed Act I of *my* story, I had not been there for the opening scenes of my mom's story either. And I judged her unfairly.

Speaking From Experience: Inspirations to Invite Healing

• **Woman Versus Food**
Several months ago, one of my online wellness subscriptions appeared in my inbox. *10 Rules to Keep the Weight Off Forever*, it read. My heart sank.

Number 1—Always eat breakfast. (Yawn.)
Number 2—Move more. (News flash?)
Number 3—Beware of "big" food. (Okay, I suppose maybe there are some folks that could bear hearing this one again.)
Number 4—Keep track. (Now I was starting to get irritated.)
By number 6, the article was recommending things like food journals, reserving indulging for "special occasions" and "following the same diet everyday."

Ugh.

Really? I thought. Are we still having this conversation? How much longer are we going to allow ourselves to participate in this woman-versus-food drama? How much longer are we going to buy into the lie that we were born just to gain and lose the same 10, 20, 50, or 100 pounds over, and over, and over again?

- **Outcomes**

The vision of an outcome can be alluring. It can also be misleading. It can look like the "perfect" family—mother, father, preppie son, girlie daughter, house with a white picket fence. It can look like wealth, fame, professional success, the winning team, or the trophy. . . .

It can also look like "skinny."

The problem with fixating on outcomes is that they are inherently filled with promise—artificial promise, that is. The vision of an outcome is a dishonest guarantee of something deeper than the outcome itself—authentic happiness, personal triumph, inner peace, even love. It is like a magnet that pulls you toward itself but never allows you to actually arrive and make meaningful contact with it. It always eludes you. It is unable to fulfill.

- **Detachment**

The reality is, the true promise of what we are searching for in the outcome is already available to us, even though we may not be available to it. The only way to find what we are truly seeking is to detach from the outcome and recognize "now" for what it is, without judgment; to be with what is, without an agenda to change it. We don't have to like it. We don't have to celebrate it. We don't have to embrace it. If we can just *be* with it without fixing, resisting, or changing it, that which has been imprisoned, that which has been the *true* object of our pursuit—authentic happiness, personal triumph, inner peace, love—becomes free. And with that freedom comes renewed access to discover a space where it may land gently, unobtrusively.

13

Verdict: Choosing Wholeness

White Noise

"Mom, do we have any chocolate?"

Once upon a time I would have known the answer without even checking. My mental inventory of all the delicious "bad" stuff had been impeccably precise. But today, that software was no longer compatible with the new computer, the healed me.

"We might," I called out. "I'll check." I rummaged through the sweets cabinet and finally found half a bag of Hershey's kisses, the ones wrapped in red, green and gold foil. Must be leftover from Christmas, I thought. It was satisfying to know I'd truly lost the storage space for this kind of hollow information.

I thought about when I used to know every detail of what sat in my kitchen cabinets as well as if I'd studied their contents to pass a national exam on them. Every bag of thin, salty, crispy, greasy, potato chips; every ounce of smooth, velvety, nutrition-less, calorie-dense chocolate; every luring baked good; every tasty leftover; all demanding that I flex my willpower muscle to full capacity. Today I wouldn't venture to begin writing a grocery list without a thorough examination of my refrigerator and cupboards . . . . because my memory no longer kept track of their contents.

I smiled to myself at the awareness of my satisfying ignorance. It was enlighteningly gratifying. It was all white noise now. Unimportant. Unnoticeable. Background. It was just . . . . *there*. And this half-eaten bag of Hershey's kisses that would have once taunted and provoked me was now as present to me as a rarely used herb from the spice rack or a five-year-old sweater I hadn't yet gotten around donating to the St. Vincent de Paul bin outside our church.

It was like that. Food was just food. All food. Watermelon, Hershey's kisses, salad, yogurt, broccoli, ice cream, pumpkin muffins, grapes, cheese, salmon, sugar cookies . . . . it was all *just* food.

It could not deem me a moral degenerate nor throne me the queen of willpower. Eating was fittingly enjoyable during the moments of consumption, but it was not euphoric bliss. It was incapable of erasing pain, healing wounds, repairing damage or filling holes. Its delicious pleasure was inherently temporary and intrinsically powerless. Always. Food was really just food again. Maybe it hadn't been "just food" since I was too little to create an entire system of crime and punishment—and self-worth—around it.

Catalyst

While I was studying to become a wellness coach, the topic of one of my nutrition classes was how to address clients suspected of having an eating disorder. I'd already been in recovery for nearly a decade, but I was still a little reserved about sharing my private history. If there was ever a safe haven to open up, this was it. The demographics of this class consisted of people who, like me, were working hard toward a common goal: transforming the collective cultural body image of womankind. My story promised to contribute valuable personal insight to the class discussion and if I could share my story here in this setting, it would prove that I had gotten past my shame and had truly forgiven myself. So I collected all the honesty I could muster into a single mass and spit it all out into the open forum.

The room was quiet. I felt a unified culmination of awareness and compassion engulfed in my secret war. A captivated professor asked me, "Do you know what it was that cured you and finally got you past all of it?"

Eating disorders are curable in about 80 percent of cases that are detected early and treated effectively.

I drew my attention inward for a brief moment. What an overwhelming irony it had all been: to have spent so many years overloading my body with vulgar amounts of that which was intended to be its very sustenance, so many years corruptly denigrating and polluting it with the very substance that ought to have been supporting its thriving, not tearing it down. It was as if in tantrum, I ungratefully and repeatedly refused an extraordinarily precious gift that had been bestowed upon me for safekeeping, and violently threw it into the face of the giver. In my hands, even grapes once held the threat of becoming poison! For every organism on this planet, the act of eating is a basic survival instinct, a law of nature. Yet I had managed to defy nature, transforming that which sustains life to that which destroys it.

I returned my attention to the unanswered question still waiting in the open air of that classroom. What cured me? I remembered my sense of urgent responsibility to heal when Travis and Taylor were born. I was driven to rescue them from any possibility of adopting my one-dimensional system of self-evaluation. There would be no chance of succeeding in this rescue mission if I wasn't fully healed myself. Children always see more than you want them to see and they learn things you don't want them to learn. I knew this firsthand—from the *other* side of the mother-child spectrum. But was motherhood the only launching pad for my healing? Did I do it for them, or did I do it for me?

Therapy had been helpful, but deep down I knew it wasn't the real cure. The day Dr. Anderson had declared me "ready," I recall a sudden panic inside me disagreeing with her unforeseen proclamation. Oh sure, my episodes were less frequent by the time I'd "graduated" from therapy, but they weren't nonexistent. Not right away. I suppose maybe therapy had a way of tilling the soil a bit, loosening the dirt so that all the ugly weeds were easier too recognize and then, pluck out, one by one.

Maybe it was a sort of fermentation of a few good seeds that happened to somehow get mixed in with all the bad ones; some messages laced with "healthy and whole" that I might have absorbed in childhood along with all the messages of "thin is beautiful and fat is ugly." And maybe even Mom had been the one to plant some of them! Maybe it was just that the good seeds had taken longer to take root and blossom. Or maybe . . . . just maybe . . . . it was ironically her brokenness that opened the window for me to find a deeper wholeness and pay it forward!

I'm pretty sure I recognized my sickness almost as soon as it showed up. I tried over and over to chase it away. It took a long time, but I guess I finally learned some way to fill myself with "right" messages over and over, even while I was submerged in so many of the "wrong" ones. So what was the true catalyst for my healing? Was there a cure or even a moment?

Then I responded with the most authentic answer afforded me.

"I think . . . . " I stopped to double-check my own truth. "I just . . . . decided." The classroom was filled with eagerly curious eyes waiting for more. "It was a *choice*." The simplicity of my response surprised even me. "The choice to heal," I continued in my own sudden leap of understanding. "When I finally *really* got that, truly understood that it was a choice . . . . I think the healing had already begun."

Choice. It's critical. Pivotal. But it's only the beginning. Waking up each morning and getting connected to that choice, attaching action and practice to it—that was the hard part. And that was also the enriching part. Right in the center of that choice was where I learned to recognize the difference between the kind of eating that feeds the body, and the other kind—the kind that feeds the destitute self, the self that believes the voice of the bully inside that tries to keep your own authentic wonderfulness a secret from you.

I remember that day well. How long ago it all suddenly felt. I hadn't had a binge-purge episode since the late 1990's, though I can't tell you the exact year. Incident-free. Isn't that what healing was about? I had felt triumphant about my achievement; confident and eager to help the expanding population of suffering women to conquer their own demons too.

But I was wrong—about my own healing, I mean. You see, in writing this book, I realized that healing is never only about what you do. It is about who you are. About deeply accepting and loving that person—the one inside—no matter where she might be along her journey. And in so doing, you begin to become capable of loving and honoring the sacredness of all life.

In my fitness work, where weight loss is generally among the top three on the almighty list of fitness goals, I have made it my trademark to stand for *inner* fitness. I have made it a practice to use carefully constructed language in my classes and with my clients that is aimed to emphasize wellness over size, strength over shape, energy over weight loss. My words are backed with depth of passion that can only exist with the aftermath of brokenness and an incremental return to wholeness. Over the years, I have desperately needed my clients to believe my words . . . . because I have desperately needed to believe them too.

Cookie Power

It was a Friday morning at 6:30 a.m., several years later in July. My cardio interval class had just ended.

"Thanks," one of the participants sighed breathlessly as she toweled off the sweat from her face and neck. "That was a great workout! I really needed that today."

I turned to face the woman whose voice I didn't recognize and smiled. "I think we all did."

"I've been in a slump," she continued. "This was the first week since New Year's that I've actually made it to the gym all five days!"

"Well congratulations then. And by the way, Happy New Year!" We chuckled and continued walking toward the lockers.

"How many days a week do *you* workout?" she asked.

"Almost everyday."

"So if I do this everyday, how long will it take me to have legs like yours?"

"Probably as long as it will take me to have *your* beautiful young skin or teeth or smile." She laughed modestly then continued to pursue her information quest. "Seriously, will an hour a day work?"

"Yes . . . . and no."

"What do you mean?"

"Yes, you'll be amazed at how just one hour a day spent reaching a little beyond your physical limits will benefit your body, and your mind, and your soul, and your energy and, and, and. And no, you won't have my legs—ever."

I noticed the playfully annoyed expression on her face saying, 'Come on, you idiot. Stop playing word-games with me. You know what I'm getting at.'

"Of course I get you," I continued. "The thing is, it's never really about redesigning our bodies. Have you ever met a single human being on this planet that was capable of doing that? And yet, we're conditioned to believe we can and should. A protein powder, a Bow-flex machine, a detox diet, a low-carb diet, a boob job, a nose job, a lap-band surgery . . . . It doesn't matter what tool we use; they all fail in the end because they don't accomplish what we don't even realize we're *really* trying to accomplish."

"Which is what, exactly?"

"We're just trying to like ourselves. And we think if we change ourselves on the outside, we'll get there. But it's not true. What really has to change is what we look through to see ourselves. We have to stop looking through the muddy stuff."

"So what's the muddy stuff?"

"All the body stuff is muddy when that's what you're looking through to see the real you. If I'm taking care of my body and making sure it's getting the stuff it needs—like food, exercise, sleep, fresh air, work, play, not to mention kindness, acceptance and compassion—then my body is just going to look like what it looks like. It's a waste of my energy to evaluate it, period. Once I free myself of that temptation to evaluate and critique my body, I get to feel all the real living and being that's always been available to me."

"Okay, I get it. My balance is just all off lately."

"Do you know why?"

"Work mostly. It's too busy. Too stressful. There's always another meeting to fit in." In a brief flashback to my years working at the insurance company, I instantly related. "And they always bring in boxes of cookies and pastries from the bakery downstairs in our building."

"You have a bakery right in your building?" I was beginning to realize it was time to lighten up and play the commiseration game. "You need a weapon, girl!"

"Yeah. I need a triple shot of willpower . . . . and about three more months of classes like that one."

"No. You need a much more powerful weapon than willpower. You need forgiveness." Her blankness told me to elaborate. "We make it such a crime to enjoy a little guilty pleasure. What's so awful about it? You're active. The cookie's probably only about 200 calories. You can work that off in fifteen minutes!" Possibly a mild exaggeration, but it was to serve a greater good.

"The problem is, I never stop at one."

"That's because of the guilt. When you tell yourself it's bad to have *any*, but then you have one anyway, you feel like you've done something wrong. That's the guilt. If it's so *wrong* you're going to feel guilty even *looking* at a cookie."

Preposterous. Who could feel guilty *looking*? But it was true. I could see the recognition of this very accurate reality in her eyes. Looking meant considering. Considering meant inner dialogue. Inner dialogue always escalated to inner debating. And that translated to win or lose. Her versus herself. A guaranteed loss either way. Then she would slap herself on the wrist and tell herself how weak she'd been. I'd seen it. I'd lived it.

"We *give* the cookie all the power. On one hand, we allow ourselves to drool over the prospect of a measly thirty seconds of what we convince ourselves will be the most luscious pleasure we've ever experienced."

"Oh my God, it is! You should see the stuff this bakery sells." I could taste the cookie coming to life in her eyes as the retrieval of the experience brought it into her present.

"On the other hand, we let eating the cookie cause us so much remorse it can ruin our whole day! Is thirty seconds of pleasure really worth two hours—or maybe even two *days*—of remorse?"

"Damn cookie power!" We laughed.

"Think about it. Who really has the power?"

"Me."

"Then don't give it away to a harmless cookie—*either* way. Eat it and *enjoy* it for the thirty seconds it's in your mouth and move on to something else without remorse. *Or* don't eat it. But don't then waste the choice to *not* eat it by torturing yourself with lustful yearnings and visions of it. Mobilize your *own* power."

"Rah-rah! I'm going to win the next cookie fight!"

"Of course you will . . . . whether you eat it or not."

Speaking From Experience: Inspirations to Invite Healing

• Goals and Dreams

Not too long ago I attended a talk at one of my career conferences where the speaker discussed the difference between goals and dreams. Goals, he said, are attached to actions in our control. Dreams are attached to outcomes, not actions, and are not in our control.

As you might imagine, transposing this distinction to the context of body image was a seamless application for me. For twenty-two years, I had treated becoming the "me" of my imagination as if it were a goal, when it had actually always been a dream.

Fixating on dreams—those images that live in our heads disguised as the promise of what is possible—usually promotes anguish, despair, and powerlessness, but shifting the focus to that which truly *is* in our control promotes empowerment. The shape and size of the body, no matter what we are brainwashed to believe, is never entirely in our control. To fixate on that outcome depletes essential energy from the actions that really work, *with* nature instead of against it, in co-creating our personal unique ideal.

• Control

Eating disorders have that word "control" written all over them. I must admit that until recently, the relationship between eating disorders and control never completely resonated with me. While I've never doubted that a perceived need to control outcomes could play into eating disorders in general, for me it always seemed to have a lot more to do with my perception of self-inadequacy than some theoretical need for control.

Though literature on the topic of Diabulimia is still a bit sparse, the research I've seen so far often suggests some pretty specific approaches to rehabilitation. Urgent messages such as, "Take action immediately," "Question your child daily," "Monitor her blood sugars yourself," are likely to appear in a majority of articles targeted to parents who suspect their diabetic child may be dealing with Diabulimia.

Where's the control here? It's being imposed externally. In situations where control may already be somewhat fragile, my fear is that this sort of aggressive removal of autonomy threatens not only to be counterproductive, but also to exacerbate the severity of an illness that may be mustering up intensity as it is.

• Healed?

While external control may indeed reform pathological behaviors that impair *physical* wellbeing and may potentially deem a Diabulimia sufferer "recovered," is this really what it means to be healed? Is true healing only about reforming *behaviors?* Is living a life of health and wholeness about conquering only those demons that are damaging to the *body?* I suspect such advice may have missed the mark on a much deeper level.

Authentic and complete healing requires courage to "go there," to tear through everything that stands in the way of that padlocked door in the basement of the soul, and then taking the risk to unlock it and look deep into the eyes of whatever stands there.

This is the source of illness. This is what lies *beneath* noxious behavior. Until we confront *this* demon, healing is incomplete and can only be on the surface.

14

Paying It Forward

Feedback Loop

Once every three hours or so, I imagine there's got to be a mother somewhere in the world who is lucky enough to finally strike gold—to be honored with one of those rare gems of motherhood: a virtual pat on the back that comes unexpectedly in the shape of something especially noble or principled that one of her children says or does. It's not necessarily a big momentous something, but it can be. More often though, it's the tiniest clue that the really important stuff, the stuff of hard-earned life lessons, the ubiquitous mantra that has come to underscore every act of parenting in which she engages, has actually landed in the right spot.

Travis approached me tentatively one night after dinner to ask permission to dye his hair black and red. He was around 13 or 14 and had blossomed into a handsome teenager with medium brown hair. Of course I preferred his natural color, but there was no harm in allowing him to play a little with his appearance, so I consented.

When Taylor got wind of it, she was appalled. "Why is he trying to be so . . . . so . . . . *goth?*" she objected. "UGH!!" But confident in her own ability to influence him, she was determined to steer him away from this "mistake."

A few days later, I learned of her nonsuccess in changing Travis' mind. I reminded her that when she was five, she used to like dressing like a boy. I had been a girlie-girl my entire life and had been so looking forward to dressing her in pinks and frills, weave fancy ribbons into her little blonde curls. But I knew even though she was only five, it was more important for me to put my personal inclination for pastels and lace aside to allow her to express herself in a way that matched *her* vision. The tomboyish image hadn't changed who she was; it allowed her to explore the possibilities of who she wanted to become—in *her* time.

"Travis needs the same freedom now," I pointed out. "I don't need to think it looks good and neither do you. He needs to choose for himself which *Travis* he wants to put out there for people to see." Then in my effort to elicit some support for her brother I added, "We all play around a little with our look before we settle into one we really like for a while. If we didn't, fashions would never change."

"But Mom . . . . what if he hates it? It's so . . . . weird. No one is born with streaks of black and red hair. It's not natural."

"When we change our hair or our clothes, or some other thing about our image, we're just saying something about how we want the world to see us. If changing his hair color is part of that statement, he has the right to make it, no matter who likes it or doesn't like it." Her body language told me that tolerance for her brother's fashion sense would be far from immediate.

Russ wasn't thrilled about the idea of Travis dyeing his hair either, but we had both done our homework and we wanted to believe we were ready for these legendary teenage whims. "Just another phase," we said often. And we both felt it was important for his developing sense of self to give him the green light, regardless of whether we agreed with his choice of color.

Russ is an exceptional dad. He listens to his children and hears what they need, not just what they say. When he feels any uncertainty about his gut reaction, he simply embraces silence. And then he embraces the true art of parenting—partnership entwined with openness. Open-mindedness doesn't come easy for Russ. He has definite opinions about some things. But he works hard at it. He also understands that when you push too hard in one direction, the other side pushes back even harder.

So one night he looked for an opening with Travis to engage in some of this "*not* pushing." He'd been waiting and watching for this moment so he was quick to recognize it when it arrived. And together he and Travis sat on our handsome son's bed laughing at something on the computer. I didn't know what it was (probably something on YouTube), but I was comforted by the laughter so I went to bed. That night my not-so-little boy proved that he was right on track for becoming a man of inner strength, individuality and character.

"Why do you want to dye your hair black and red anyway?" Russ asked casually. "What are you trying to put out there about yourself?"

"I don't know," Travis answered honestly. "I guess I just want to see how I look." And then, as if to provide his dad with that tiny morsel of reassurance he intuitively seemed to know was needed in the moment, "Dad . . . . it's only hair. It's not going to change anything about who I am on the inside."

There it was—the line—the one axiom through this entire flirtation with typical teenage thirst for independence and nonconformity that would become a precursor to the sensitive and courageous human being my son would come to be. All that he would one day become was already inside him, waiting to ripen.

My eighth grade son already knew what it had taken me a lifetime to integrate: the important stuff is the stuff you can't see on the outside.

Travis never did end up dying his hair red and black. I never asked him what changed his mind. In the end, it didn't really matter.

*   *   *

My mother-in-law loves my kids nearly as much as Russ and I do. Even today Travis and Taylor are the nucleus of most of our conversations. I suppose at her age, a daily walk down Memory Lane becomes a necessary part of your morning exercise routine.

"She is so gorgeous!"

My mother-in-law was referring to Taylor. She was right. I don't know if it's the glistening blonde curls, the sparkle in her translucent blue eyes, or the modest smile that has a way of saying, "Life is just plain awesome!" but Taylor is definitely one of those girls who turns heads everywhere she goes.

"I remember when she was little I used to tell her every time I saw her how beautiful she was," my mother-in-law continued. "One day she just turned to me and said, 'Grammy, it's more important to be beautiful on the *inside* than on the outside.' She sounded so cute and so smart."

"How old was she?" I asked my mother-in-law when her delightful moment of reminiscence took a short pause. I was mentally piecing together where this adorable little snippet fit into the bigger timeline.

"Well, it was when I was taking care of them, so she must have been about three or four."

A perfect fit. I knew exactly where it had come from. It was just around the time I'd finished my sessions with Dr. Anderson. I must admit that if an adult had spoken those same words, it would border on cliché, but coming from Taylor's four-year-old mouth it had been anything but. For her it was just the truth—because Mom said so. Even hearing the story through my mother-in-law's retelling I could hear my own voice.

I instantly was reminded of a similar conversation I'd had with Taylor, probably around the same time.

"What do you think is more important to me?" I had asked her. "That you are pretty, smart, or happy?"

Her answer had required no deliberation at all. "Happy." Her confidence in responding (not to mention the response itself) left me feeling reassured that even though I was not going to get through this parenting game error-free, at least the "right" messages were making greater impact than any of the "wrong" ones that might occasionally slip out. (I guess every now and then, even I was capable of hitting a grand slam!)

By her sophomore year in high school, Taylor was beginning to demonstrate the kind of leadership potential to which highly educated adults of academia and well-trained professionals of corporate America aspire. She radiated a refreshing balance between confidence and humility, courage and composure; neither engorged with self-importance nor suffocated by self-doubt. She showed occasional and moderate healthy attention to her physical appearance, but did not mistake it for the self inside her. She seemed to have just the right amount of everything—respect for diversity, the planet, humankind; authentic gratitude for life and love; a special compassion for animals, the elderly, people with special needs. I saw it, but I wasn't the only one. Her teachers saw it; her guidance counselors saw it; other moms saw it. By her junior year, Taylor was elected into the 2009 class of *Tomorrow 25*, a *Time* magazine and Bentley College-sponsored leadership forum for high school juniors around the world who displayed outstanding potential to become a "leader of tomorrow."

I felt oh so proud of my wonderful budding daughter, but more than pride for her, I felt joy for her. She was an exquisite plant, now growing into all of the beauty that had always been waiting to ripen from within her. And I was just one of a multitude of gardeners blessed with the sweet responsibility of cultivating the soil in which she would continue to grow and flourish. As her mother, I was charged with many important tasks, some which would remain under my jurisdiction forever.

I found it warmly reassuring and heartening to witness my daughter, and more specifically, where she stood. To view it against the backdrop of where I had stood at her age was respite for my soul. She faced practically zero danger of ever walking through the dark places I had seen.

How could this be *my* daughter? Me! The one who used to hate herself so much she would deliberately allow herself to practically die—over and over and over again—trying to become someone else! How could someone like that produce someone like *this*?

But I knew the truth, at least one of many truths: Taylor was who she was partly *because* of the places I had traveled. Spending time in the center of those ugly places had made me determined to install in Taylor's heart, a genuine honor and gratitude for the person *inside* the gorgeous young woman she had become. My own journey had forewarned me of the cultural pollution of body obsession she would inevitably encounter. But I had armed her against it, not by avoiding or denying it; by authentically responding to it; by calling both of us out on the misdirected thinking that could lure you into that shallow space; even by acknowledging my own temptation to still go there now and then.

Should I presume to own credit for the triumph of Travis' and Taylor's successes in life? Not a chance. Did I get to celebrate them with them? Absolutely. Am I now allowed to take part in enjoying the fruit of this beautiful garden that I have devoted so many years to pruning and watering? You betcha!

And if either Travis or Taylor should happen to bump into heartache, anguish, rejection, or that horrible feeling of failure or self-doubt, I will be right here beside them to help pull out the weeds and trim away the dried up leaves to make way for the off-shoots of rebirth. I do hope that when that happens, I'll remember to celebrate that too, to remind all of us that hurting almost always means you are about to grow.

As desperately and aggressively as I had hunted motherhood down, I once secretly had feared I might not be its best candidate, not because I didn't recognize the criteria of good parenting, but because I might involuntarily propagate the cycle of damage from within the center of my own brokenness. But my children were teaching me, in big ways and in small ways, that history doesn't repeat itself. Not really.

Second Chance

It was March 31, 2008 when the headlines in the Health section of *The Boston Globe* called out to me in decibels: "*Dying to be thin.*" I sat down with my oatmeal and morning coffee and read about a girl who had died from the relationship between her eating disorder and diabetes.

"She calls it black magic," the article began. "Every time her jeans start feeling tight, she skips a few doses of the insulin she needs to treat her diabetes. The pounds slip off—but there's a price. . . . "

I studied the black and white portrait on that newspaper page. The stranger in the photo had boney elbows and sad sunken-in eyes. But it wasn't just a picture in the paper. It was a real person, with real family, and real friends—relationships that had probably been cheated out of countless moments, and replaced with food orgies, projectile puke sessions with the nearest toilet, and regular police-escorted trips to the E.R.

The girl's gaunt hollow eyes took me to another time—a time when the heaviness of shame and failure repeatedly anchored me to the sterile coldness of hospital bed after hospital bed and held me captive there each time; when violent oppressive thirst regularly insisted its way into me, sucking every last molecule of aliveness from my body; when even breathing was such an intolerable movement against my dry trachea that it triggered violent gag reflexes, and inescapable explosions of vomiting, until there was nothing left inside me other than the toxins that took the place of healthy body fluids.

The newspaper lay on the table next to where I was eating my oatmeal. The stranger with the boney elbows looked up at me. I looked into her sad sunken-in eyes, and at once, I knew her. Knew who she was, what she was feeling. I wanted so badly to hug the sad lost girl on that page and fix all that was broken inside her, help her to learn all that she really was. But it was too late for that.

For a long moment that seemed to have no beginning or end, I allowed myself to disappear into the world I imagined once belonged to this young girl. Without meaning to, I began inventing details of her short life; details that resembled a life I'd already tucked away forever.

And I knew at once—this girl was not a stranger at all.

I suddenly reawakened to the ordinariness of morning, now progressing in a steady rhythm around me. I hadn't noticed the strain of stifled tears that had begun to brew behind the brim of my eye sockets. A throbbing compassion started to swell inside me—for the stranger, and for the child I used to be. I sat with that compassion for a minute or so before determination moved in to take its place, filling up all the space inside me with a renewed sense of purpose, a purpose bigger than anything that had ever before occupied that space. And I spoke, almost aloud, with a bittersweet blend of regret and gratitude.

Thank you God, I cried, my silent words choking me from the back of my throat. *I'm SO sorry. I was KILLING myself all those years. You gave me this precious gift of life, and I treated it with complete disregard and irreverence. I abused and mutilated it and risked everything you allowed me to have. How could I have ever maltreated such a treasure? Please forgive me God. . . .*

I buried my forehead into my hands and glanced down at my steaming bowl of oatmeal sprinkled with cinnamon and chopped walnuts. Walnuts, I thought. Ten years ago I wouldn't have dared to come within two feet of these nourishing gems of monounsaturated fat.

And God? I continued in silent prayer. *Thank you for the second chance. The chance to make things right. To use the wretchedness of those agonizing years for something meaningful. I get it now. I really do. I am not so sure I deserve this second chance, but thank you for it. I won't blow it.*

The kids were now spilling their backpacks, sports bags and musical instruments into the car so I promptly cleared my dishes and dropped Travis and Taylor off at school. Then I was off to teach my second fitness class of the morning.

Morning's Symphony

I am a morning person. To me these first few moments of daybreak have somehow always stood for possibility, renewal, starting over. I love the rich robust aroma of freshly brewed coffee and the colorful peeks of sunrise hiding between the branches just beyond my porch. But my favorite part of morning is awaking to the sweet music of distant bird dialogue. It is Morning's Symphony.

On summer mornings I bring my breakfast and coffee onto our screened-in porch just to get a little closer to that music.

A few years ago I was sitting in my usual spot at the table on the porch, drinking up all that the day's first moments had to offer me. The branches were in great need of trimming, but I liked them this way. They were much closer to me in their overgrown state and enclosed the porch like Nature's canopy. I was especially alert on this particular morning, intentionally watchful. A tiny yellow bird caught my eye. I took a sip of my coffee and followed the bird as it danced cheerfully, from one branch to another. I watched it nibble on an oak leaf (though I can't be sure whether it was nibbling on the leaf itself or an insect *on* the leaf). It was so simple and carefree and beautiful. Not just the bird; the whole scene. It looked like something you'd see at the beginning of a schmaltzy romance movie or something. I was completely enchanted with the moment.

Birds are in complete harmony with life, I kept thinking. What kind of absurdity would it be to witness a robin red breast in inner turmoil over having just eaten one too many grubs, or a cardinal resolving to fly the entire east coast to work off an overindulgent feast of worms just to prevent itself from an inevitable thickening rump beneath its tail feathers. I chuckled almost aloud at the preposterousness of my thoughts.

Birds listen to the commands of one leader, I thought: Nature. They don't debate or deliberate or resist or even choose. Nature tells them when to sing, when to fly, when to nest, and when to refuel. And they obey. Always. Birds don't *plan* who they want to be. They don't *decide* to change what Nature has made them. They are who they are. And they accept what Nature offers them unconditionally. I don't think anyone would call them fierce creatures, yet they are among the freest. No car is too fast, no tower is too high, and no river is too wide to prevent them from flying wherever it is that Nature is calling them to be.

I sipped the last bit of coffee from my Starbucks mug. The sun was now beginning to cast hues of orange and pink over the tree-lined horizon. The trees surrounding me were now practically dancing with aliveness of the full bird-orchestra for sunrise's coda. There was so much going on up there. Noticing was no longer something I was doing; it was happening to me. I was no longer listening for the music; it just filled the air around me. I stopped watching the graceful choreography amidst the branches; my soul just became a part of it. The fragrance of moistened earth was no longer separate from me; I was drinking it into me with every breath. Every cubic inch of morning was one unified masterpiece of hope and possibility.

Now I'm no Henry David Thoreau, but this morning, this space—well, it really was magnificent. If you've never just sat beneath the largeness of Creation before, without doing or even thinking, I strongly recommend it. Wisdom and perspective have a unique way of finding you. But you can't look for them. And don't expect them to land every time. They're unpredictable. Just be open and awake. When you're ready, they'll know exactly where to find you.

The yellow bird was still nibbling, jumping, flapping, fluttering . . . . and nibbling again. Life for birds was pretty simple. We could really learn something from these creatures. Maybe learning to listen a little closer to Nature could make life simple for us too.

I opened the sliding doors to the kitchen and grabbed my laptop. Returning to my spot at the table on the porch, I lay it down and opened a new Word document.

And the music of that morning would become the soundtrack for the birth of my memoir.

New Purpose

When I decided to write a book about coming through the other side of my eating disorder, I took it to be my calling. This is what I was meant to do, my unique contribution to humankind. Writing a book that might make a difference for other sufferers would dissolve any residual shame surrounding that epic struggle once and for all, even make it worth something meaningful. As it turns out, writing this book was much bigger than the book.

In the process of writing and rewriting, I found myself returning to another time, first looking back, then looking inside—deep inside. Mostly I suppose, I was looking for the purest honesty I could find. As I read every word that spilled out of me from a place that had been safely padlocked in the basement of my heart for what felt like eons, it was as though I finally could see the landscape beyond my bedroom window for the first time— the branches of the tall oak above, the cracks in the driveway below—scenery that had been there all along. I read my very own words, and really heard them. Only now, I heard more than words; I heard what was behind them and inside them. To be honest, I now think I was walking through the center of the most important part of healing, *as* I was writing this book, not before.

After I wrote my first draft, the literary agent with whom I was working at the time encouraged me to write a more prescriptive manuscript—you know, one of those self-help books. I resisted the idea. Who was I to presume the expertise to plot the course through anyone else's stormy waters? Heck, I barely felt competent to navigate through my own. No two journeys are the same, I thought. They may intersect, parallel or mirror each other, but they are never exactly the same. Having arrived here in this place of healing and renewal hardly qualified me as an authority on the subject. The steps that led to this place were not part of some well-thought-out, clearly defined methodology. They were messy, complicated. But though the steps of recovery showed up in a variety of shapes, they all shared one thing in common: At the core of each one, stood choice and openness.

For sure, if I could give just one piece of advice about healing, not just from Diabulimia, but the bruises we bear from stumbling through *any* of life's darkness, it would be to listen, *really* listen—with guttural honesty and unobstructed openness—to the clues that have been hidden specifically in that darkness for us to discover, and look for the pieces of Truth illuminated and then make the *choice* to do whatever healing asks, no matter how messy or scary.

The Distance

Metaphors. What is it about them that I love so much? I guess it's that they have a way of opening my mind to a new way of seeing. They put things on a completely different plane, in fact. Sure, they crystallize and clarify, but it's more than that. They are musical, poetic. They turn words into art. I love them. Love to read them, hear them, create them and use them. Even the cliché ones. So go ahead. Pick one: spiraling down a bottomless hole; standing on the wrong side of a brick wall; imprisoned by the handcuffs of Perfection Hell.

Whichever one you choose, I'd beaten it. I'd climbed out that hole, dismantled that wall, escaped that hell. But as monumental as it had been, I couldn't really pinpoint the exact moment of this Olympic victory. I suppose I could come up with several milestones on the way to the Gold Medal (there I go again . . . . always the incurable metaphor junkie), but the truth is I lived through so many false grand finales that it's nearly impossible to isolate a single pivotal moment of healing.

The important thing is there were many times I tried to climb out of that hole and fell to the bottom. Each time I fell, that bottom was a little lower than the last, but it didn't stop me from trying to regain my footing to make my way out of that hole. I slammed into that brick wall countless times before I figured out it had to come down one brick at a time. And I turned many different keys before finding one that would unlock those handcuffs.

Here's the truth: As fearful as I once had been about inheriting some imaginary "I-Give-Up" gene, there was a force far more powerful in me than that fear the whole time—hope. And boy, was it stubborn! I just kept deciding, trying, failing, and trying again. Hope or fear? I guess in the end, hope wins.

Now and then, I look back at the jagged footpath of successes and failings as if viewing my personal scrapbook. I turn the page, and sometimes I'm struck by an unexpected view—a breathtaking view actually—much more amazing than the vision of one single catalyst of healing. It is the vision of immeasurable length between where I once stood and where I stand now. I don't always see it, so when I do, I so want to celebrate. But it isn't just standing here, in this place where I'm all healed and whole again, that I want to celebrate. It's not just about where I am now. It's all the space *between* then and now. I want to celebrate the *distance*.

Today I see imperfection and rejoice. Hooray for imperfections! They're gorgeous! Today I see "real" and give it a great big bear hug. Today I live inside a peaceful space; peace itself has taken up permanent residence inside me. And I know for sure this treasure is mine, not in spite of my journey, but because of it.

I suppose the true value of anything in life, whether it shows up as deep timeless joy or an epic medical tragedy, is best appraised not by its residue of drama but by its fruits. My inner journey is undeniably the longest and hardest distance I've ever walked, but the journey itself has everything to do with who I am today. And I would take that walk all over again. You see, somewhere in the darkness of those miles, I know that I have found the greatest treasure a person can find: a deep connection with true Selfhood. It was there all along.

Speaking From Experience: Inspirations to Invite Healing

• Toxic Promises

In simplest terms, weight loss—regardless of the strategy to achieve it—is a promise to self. When a breach of promise is committed, it is hurtful to the beneficiary of the promise. When that beneficiary is the self, it is a violation of the most deeply personal kind, and the sting is fundamentally profound. It is the ultimate betrayal.

The very moment a commitment to self exists in thought form, it is real. Whether the commitment holds value or toxicity is irrelevant to the reality of its presence. In either case, a broken promise begets only one possible verdict: guilty. When a crime is committed there is always a consequence, whether it is imposed from some external source or from within.

• Duality

Making toxic promises can become habitual and often unconscious. It sets up an inner duality of self versus self and fuels perpetual inner conflict. On one hand there is the "promise-maker self" who deals only in absolutes and is incapable of justifying or tolerating broken promises of any kind, even toxic ones ("I will not eat anything but lettuce all day!"). This self recognizes the promise as a valuable entity but doesn't distinguish whether its content is nourishing or toxic. She is therefore morally bound to keep the promise lest the beneficiary be dishonored. In a roundabout way, it's an odd gesture of self-respect.

On the other hand, there is the self that recognizes the toxicity and is therefore compelled to break it. Each aspect of self is acting according to its assigned code of ethics and within the limitations of its own inner wiring.

• Whole Again

If we call upon our *intention* to become conscious, we give ourselves access to something truly amazing. Habitualness is replaced with purposefulness. We become capable of breaking apart the anatomy of a promise and evaluating its worthiness before "signing the contract." Toxic promises begin to fade and the cycle of inner duality is broken. The promises we make to ourselves become nourishing, not to outcomes, but to the journey. And in that original intention to become conscious, we have given ourselves the opportunity to become whole again.

15

Shopping Resurrected

Another Green Dress

I have always loved clothes shopping. What woman doesn't? Shoes, bags, dresses, accessories . . . . What a fun way to luxuriate—not to mention strip your bank account. I think I have finally figured out its real attraction. It's all about the illusions. We're drawn to them. Fashion is its own art where individuality and creativity fuse through cleverly designed illusion to produce a powerfully effective placebo for self-esteem.

Recently, I went to the mall to buy a dress to wear for Easter. There's something especially enticing to me about dress shopping in the spring. The styles have a way of foreshadowing the lush season of aliveness approaching the cycle of nature's landscape.

I chose a few attractive styles from the *New Arrivals* rack of Ann Taylor and carried them into the fitting room with me. I slid a green dress off the hanger and slipped it over my head, smoothing out the wrinkles as I pulled it over the rest of my body. Then I carefully scrutinized its effect on the image in the full-view mirror.

Today, thirty-some-odd years after that shockingly revelatory day in front of my bedroom mirror, that tight Kelly green polyester fabric imprisoning my body like a vise, I inspected my reflection with different eyes. Today's eyes had already stopped looking for perfection. They knew that there is nothing beautiful or even interesting about it. It is boring and contrived and artificial. But *imperfection* is extraordinary, unique, organic, and real. And it is the only size that honest beauty comes in. All you have to do is look at a sunset sky. Some of the most inspiring ones I've beheld have had a few clouds leftover from the afternoon. I think somehow it's the clouds themselves that give the sky its color variations. *That's* what I find breathtaking!

The green dress I saw in today's mirror didn't show me ugly or fat like that thirty-five-year-ago dress had. Today's green dress just showed the *real* me.

I tucked the price tags inside the sleeve and neck so that I could better imagine this dress as mine. The dress hugged my waistline and draped slightly away from my hips. It almost made my five-feet-two-inch frame appear somewhat taller. Just another illusion, I thought. The subtle lines of this dress were skillfully sewn together to create smooth curves and graceful stylish flow. The light cotton fabric was a vibrant tone of jade green with subtle hints of opal white and creamy yellow, creating a vague floral impression. Very springy, I thought. I draped it over my arm and sauntered up to the cashier.

I once looked in the mirror and saw flaws and imperfection. Today I see much more.

Speaking From Experience: Inspirations to Invite Healing

• **For You**
I want to thank you for inviting my story into your life. For one reason or another, you opened this book and allowed me to share my journey with you. Perhaps it was that something in its title held the promise of connecting to a piece of your own truth. Or maybe you are a parent of someone you suspect might be grappling with Diabulimia and you wondered if my story might offer you a tiny window into her experience. Or it could be simply that you find healing stories inspiring.

Whatever your reason, these short sections at the end of each chapter of my memoir have been written for you. They have been specifically designed to engender personal reflection and, for some of you, to become just one possible source of enlightenment, connection, and exploration along your own journey.

• **The Gift of Difficulty**
When I was originally asked to write these segments, their suggested title was to be "SPEAKING FROM EXPERIENCE: TIPS TO MAKE THE

JOURNEY EASIER." While I embraced the idea of supplementing my memoir with text that held potential for practical use, I labored and vacillated over the word "easier."

I considered all kinds of ideas about what kinds of things to include, but as long as I mused, as hard as I tried, I simply could not find a workable angle for that word "easier." From where I stood, not only was "easier" not possible, it would have been incapable of giving me all I have received.

I am where I am today *because* it was difficult. And though I cannot take away challenges that may await you, I can promise you that there are always gems hidden at their core, gems hidden underneath every difficulty. The gems are the very reason difficulty shows up.

• What Angels Look Like

I believe that God sends us only angels, or if you prefer, that life sends us only teachers. Sometimes they look like light; sometimes they look like darkness. They can make life easier or smoother or clearer or more wonderful; and they can make life hard or painful— just to create a clearing for new richness to enter.

I have learned that healing from life's injuries is not an event or an occurrence; it is a process. Before we can begin to heal, we must ask the injury what it came to teach, and we must be ready for the answer when it comes. Whatever we refuse to see and feel and learn will never walk away, so we must be ready to see and feel and learn the truths that pain embodies. They are the truths that may be heard in the resounding echo of a blaring "aha moment," and sometimes they are truths that can only be heard in the wise whisper of stillness.

Epilogue

The Number Police

I'd love to be able to tell you that I never give any thought whatsoever to body weight, calories, or fat grams anymore, but I'd be lying. Truth is, those disapproving little Number Police still show up now and then, and when they do, they use every trick in the book to get inside my head. They seem to have a sixth sense for knowing which door is easiest to break down, and a sixth sense for choosing the worst possible time to hang out on the other side of it—like when I've put too many things in the in-box of life and happen to be cutting a batch of brownies. I can always tell when those ugly little guys are lurking, ready to pounce, just watching for their moment to break in. Most of the time though, they fail.

I suppose the threat of using food to fill something other than my stomach is always looming in the distance somewhere. But even if that does happen—if something does happen to cross my lips sort of unconsciously—I don't binge anymore; I just eat. And I don't purge; I just let being alive use up its own calories without bothering to calculate or expel them. And being alive? Well sometimes that includes having one of those dreaded fat days. But I get through it. Not around it, mind you—*through* it. I take a long hard look in the mirror and remind myself that what I see is not ugly fat; it's beautiful stored-up energy whose purpose is to serve me if I need it. Or, if that doesn't work, I slip on the baggy jeans for the day, check in with God, search out the pieces of life that really mean something, and trust that the feeling will leave me in its own time. It always does—when it's ready.

I used to hope that healing would somehow just appear on my doorstep and fix me; that temptation would suddenly stop showing up all around me, or stop *being* temptation altogether; or that willpower might grow strong enough to take it over and destroy it. But healing—like everything that's *real*—doesn't arrive like that, all neatly wrapped in some fantasized box of perfection. It's more like a flawed package imbued with choice, struggle, and acceptance. It's not a prescription; it's a long, unpredictable, messy miracle with huge setbacks, tiny triumphs, and mind-blowing epiphanies.

I guess healing—real healing—is never about overcoming temptation. I guess it's never about overcoming anything. It is about knowing that it's really okay to not overcome it. And it's even okay to feel bad about not overcoming it. It's about forgiveness. Real forgiveness. The kind where you just open your hands and let whatever it was you were clinging to fall into a space where you'll never see it again. And then, you move onto the next moment. It's where forgiveness, surrender and love all intersect. Healing is *that* place.

I have a little secret to tell you, something I've only learned recently: Perfection really *does* exist! It's just that it doesn't look like what I once thought. And you know what's even more amazing? We are all perfect already! We are exactly the way we are "supposed" to be. Every single one of us!

How ironic that something as innocent as a crust of bread, a finger dipped in peanut butter, or a fresh picked tomato can be life-sustaining nourishment in one moment, and in the next, emotional, psychological, and yes, even physical poison. It's a perverse mockery of human nature.

Funny how lies become impossible to believe once you've shared space with truth. You ask yourself, 'How did I ever not see that truth before?'

I suppose I must have presumed that by losing body fat, I would some-how miraculously gain something wonderful in its place. And whatever that something wonderful was, I was ravenously hungry for it. Hungry—but not for food. I was hungry for the unshakable, unbreakable belief that I was already enough. Maybe that's all any of us are hungry for. You know, the hunger underneath all other hungers—ambition, greed, narcissism; athletic, academic or economic competitiveness; unquenchable thirst for fame, wealth, status, power, rank. And there, right at the core of it all, one single common denominator—a fundamental longing to be more than we are at this moment. Maybe the only thing any of us are hungry for is just to be enough. Right now. That's a big burden to put on food.

The Number Police still come around sometimes, but hardly ever. And when they do show up, I've learned to acknowledge them. But I don't invite them to dinner, and they never end up staying very long. The thing is, I don't think they feel very welcome anymore. You see, they're power freaks. They don't like to hang out in places where they don't get to call the shots . . . . and *I'm* in charge now, even when I feel like I'm not. They know now that the only power they have—the only power they've ever had—is the power I give them. They sometimes forget that, but I guess that's okay too.

*　　*　　*

Do you have diabetes like 25.8 million other Americans? Have you ever altered or omitted insulin in an attempt to lose weight? You are not alone! Nearly half of teen and young adult females with Type 1 Diabetes have at least considered it. But there are people who are here to help you through this journey. Don't lose your eyesight, your kidneys, your feet . . . . or your *life* to this disease. Please contact one of the organizations listed in the back of this book for support.

Resources for People with Eating Disorders

AED: Academy for Eating Disorders
111 Deer Lake Road, Suite 100
Deerfield, IL 60015
Phone: (847) 498-4274 Fax: (847) 480-9282

For ED professionals; promotes effective treatment, develops prevention initiatives, stimulates research, sponsors international conference.

ANAD: National Association of Anorexia Nervosa & Associated Disorders
Phone: (847) 831-3438

Distributes listing of therapists, hospitals, and informative materials; sponsors support groups, conferences, advocacy campaigns, research, and a crisis hotline.

Eating Disorders Coalition for Research, Policy and Action
720 7th Street NW, #300
Washington, DC 20001
Phone: (202) 543-9570, Fax: (202) 543-9570

Their mission is to advance the federal recognition of eating disorders as a public health priority.

Eating for Life Alliance
396 Washington Street, Suite 392
Wellesley, MA 02481
www.eatingforlife.org

A new Wellesley, Massachusetts-based program geared toward college students with eating disorders.

IAEDP: International Association of Eating Disorders Professionals
P.O. Box 1295
Pekin, IL 61555-1295
(800) 800-8126

A membership organization for professionals; provides certification, education, local chapters, a newsletter, and an annual symposium.

NEDA: National Eating Disorders Association
601 Stewart Street, Suite 803
Seattle, WA 98101
Phone: (206) 382-3587
Hotline: (800) 931-2237

The National Eating Disorders Association (NEDA) is the largest not-for-profit organization in the United States working to prevent eating disorders and providing treatment referrals to those suffering from anorexia, bulimia and binge eating disorders and those concerned with body image and weight issues.

Resources for People with Diabetes

American Diabetes Association
ATTN: National Call Center
1701 North Beauregard Street
Alexandria, VA 22311
Phone: 1-800-DIABETES (1-800-342-2383)

Joslin Diabetes Center
One Joslin Place
Boston, MA 02215
Phone: (617) 732-2400
(800) JOSLIN-1
(800) 567-5461
diabetes@joslin.harvard.edu

Juvenile Diabetes Research Foundation International
26 Broadway, 14th Floor
New York, NY 10004
Phone: 1-800-533-CURE (2873)
Fax: (212) 785-9595
info@jdrf.org

The Barton Center for Diabetes Education
30 Ennis Road
PO Box 356
North Oxford, MA 01537-0356
Phone: (508) 987-2056
info@bartoncenter.org

Index